Mometrix
TEST PREPARATION

AF701165

CWCN®

Exam Secrets Study Guide

Dear Future Exam Success Story

First of all, **THANK YOU** for purchasing Mometrix study materials!

Second, congratulations! You are one of the few determined test-takers who are committed to doing whatever it takes to excel on your exam. **You have come to the right place.** We developed these study materials with one goal in mind: to deliver you the information you need in a format that's concise and easy to use.

In addition to optimizing your guide for the content of the test, we've outlined our recommended steps for breaking down the preparation process into small, attainable goals so you can make sure you stay on track.

We've also analyzed the entire test-taking process, identifying the most common pitfalls and showing how you can overcome them and be ready for any curveball the test throws you.

Standardized testing is one of the biggest obstacles on your road to success, which only increases the importance of doing well in the high-pressure, high-stakes environment of test day. Your results on this test could have a significant impact on your future, and this guide provides the information and practical advice to help you achieve your full potential on test day.

Your success is our success

We would love to hear from you! If you would like to share the story of your exam success or if you have any questions or comments in regard to our products, please contact us at **800-673-8175** or **support@mometrix.com**.

Thanks again for your business and we wish you continued success!

Sincerely,
The Mometrix Test Preparation Team

Need more help? Check out our flashcards at:
http://MometrixFlashcards.com/WOCNCB

TABLE OF CONTENTS

Introduction

Thank you for purchasing this resource! You have made the choice to prepare yourself for a test that could have a huge impact on your future, and this guide is designed to help you be fully ready for test day. Obviously, it's important to have a solid understanding of the test material, but you also need to be prepared for the unique environment and stressors of the test, so that you can perform to the best of your abilities.

For this purpose, the first section that appears in this guide is the **Secret Keys**. We've devoted countless hours to meticulously researching what works and what doesn't, and we've boiled down our findings to the five most impactful steps you can take to improve your performance on the test. We start at the beginning with study planning and move through the preparation process, all the way to the testing strategies that will help you get the most out of what you know when you're finally sitting in front of the test.

We recommend that you start preparing for your test as far in advance as possible. However, if you've bought this guide as a last-minute study resource and only have a few days before your test, we recommend that you skip over the first two Secret Keys since they address a long-term study plan.

If you struggle with **test anxiety**, we strongly encourage you to check out our recommendations for how you can overcome it. Test anxiety is a formidable foe, but it can be beaten, and we want to make sure you have the tools you need to defeat it.

Secret Key #1 – Plan Big, Study Small

There's a lot riding on your performance. If you want to ace this test, you're going to need to keep your skills sharp and the material fresh in your mind. You need a plan that lets you review everything you need to know while still fitting in your schedule. We'll break this strategy down into three categories.

Information Organization

Start with the information you already have: the official test outline. From this, you can make a complete list of all the concepts you need to cover before the test. Organize these concepts into groups that can be studied together, and create a list of any related vocabulary you need to learn so you can brush up on any difficult terms. You'll want to keep this vocabulary list handy once you actually start studying since you may need to add to it along the way.

Time Management

Once you have your set of study concepts, decide how to spread them out over the time you have left before the test. Break your study plan into small, clear goals so you have a manageable task for each day and know exactly what you're doing. Then just focus on one small step at a time. When you manage your time this way, you don't need to spend hours at a time studying. Studying a small block of content for a short period each day helps you retain information better and avoid stressing over how much you have left to do. You can relax knowing that you have a plan to cover everything in time. In order for this strategy to be effective though, you have to start studying early and stick to your schedule. Avoid the exhaustion and futility that comes from last-minute cramming!

Study Environment

The environment you study in has a big impact on your learning. Studying in a coffee shop, while probably more enjoyable, is not likely to be as fruitful as studying in a quiet room. It's important to keep distractions to a minimum. You're only planning to study for a short block of time, so make the most of it. Don't pause to check your phone or get up to find a snack. It's also important to **avoid multitasking**. Research has consistently shown that multitasking will make your studying dramatically less effective. Your study area should also be comfortable and well-lit so you don't have the distraction of straining your eyes or sitting on an uncomfortable chair.

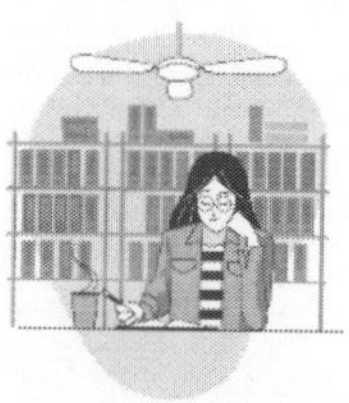

The time of day you study is also important. You want to be rested and alert. Don't wait until just before bedtime. Study when you'll be most likely to comprehend and remember. Even better, if you know what time of day your test will be, set that time aside for study. That way your brain will be used to working on that subject at that specific time and you'll have a better chance of recalling information.

Finally, it can be helpful to team up with others who are studying for the same test. Your actual studying should be done in as isolated an environment as possible, but the work of organizing the information and setting up the study plan can be divided up. In between study sessions, you can discuss with your teammates the concepts that you're all studying and quiz each other on the details. Just be sure that your teammates are as serious about the test as you are. If you find that your study time is being replaced with social time, you might need to find a new team.

Secret Key #2 – Make Your Studying Count

You're devoting a lot of time and effort to preparing for this test, so you want to be absolutely certain it will pay off. This means doing more than just reading the content and hoping you can remember it on test day. It's important to make every minute of study count. There are two main areas you can focus on to make your studying count.

Retention

It doesn't matter how much time you study if you can't remember the material. You need to make sure you are retaining the concepts. To check your retention of the information you're learning, try recalling it at later times with minimal prompting. Try carrying around flashcards and glance at one or two from time to time or ask a friend who's also studying for the test to quiz you.

To enhance your retention, look for ways to put the information into practice so that you can apply it rather than simply recalling it. If you're using the information in practical ways, it will be much easier to remember. Similarly, it helps to solidify a concept in your mind if you're not only reading it to yourself but also explaining it to someone else. Ask a friend to let you teach them about a concept you're a little shaky on (or speak aloud to an imaginary audience if necessary). As you try to summarize, define, give examples, and answer your friend's questions, you'll understand the concepts better and they will stay with you longer. Finally, step back for a big picture view and ask yourself how each piece of information fits with the whole subject. When you link the different concepts together and see them working together as a whole, it's easier to remember the individual components.

Finally, practice showing your work on any multi-step problems, even if you're just studying. Writing out each step you take to solve a problem will help solidify the process in your mind, and you'll be more likely to remember it during the test.

Modality

Modality simply refers to the means or method by which you study. Choosing a study modality that fits your own individual learning style is crucial. No two people learn best in exactly the same way, so it's important to know your strengths and use them to your advantage.

For example, if you learn best by visualization, focus on visualizing a concept in your mind and draw an image or a diagram. Try color-coding your notes, illustrating them, or creating symbols that will trigger your mind to recall a learned concept. If you learn best by hearing or discussing information, find a study partner who learns the same way or read aloud to yourself. Think about how to put the information in your own words. Imagine that you are giving a lecture on the topic and record yourself so you can listen to it later.

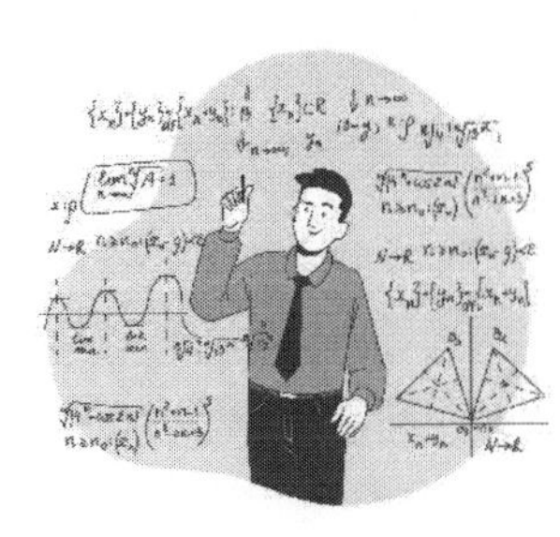

For any learning style, flashcards can be helpful. Organize the information so you can take advantage of spare moments to review. Underline key words or phrases. Use different colors for different categories. Mnemonic devices (such as creating a short list in which every item starts with the same letter) can also help with retention. Find what works best for you and use it to store the information in your mind most effectively and easily.

Secret Key #3 – Practice the Right Way

Your success on test day depends not only on how many hours you put into preparing, but also on whether you prepared the right way. It's good to check along the way to see if your studying is paying off. One of the most effective ways to do this is by taking practice tests to evaluate your progress. Practice tests are useful because they show exactly where you need to improve. Every time you take a practice test, pay special attention to these three groups of questions:

- The questions you got wrong
- The questions you had to guess on, even if you guessed right
- The questions you found difficult or slow to work through

This will show you exactly what your weak areas are, and where you need to devote more study time. Ask yourself why each of these questions gave you trouble. Was it because you didn't understand the material? Was it because you didn't remember the vocabulary? Do you need more repetitions on this type of question to build speed and confidence? Dig into those questions and figure out how you can strengthen your weak areas as you go back to review the material.

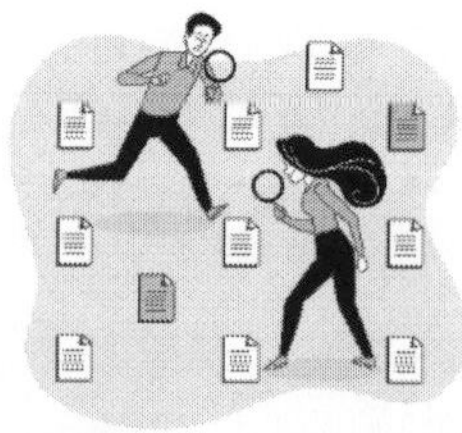

Additionally, many practice tests have a section explaining the answer choices. It can be tempting to read the explanation and think that you now have a good understanding of the concept. However, an explanation likely only covers part of the question's broader context. Even if the explanation makes perfect sense, **go back and investigate** every concept related to the question until you're positive you have a thorough understanding.

As you go along, keep in mind that the practice test is just that: practice. Memorizing these questions and answers will not be very helpful on the actual test because it is unlikely to have any of the same exact questions. If you only know the right answers to the sample questions, you won't be prepared for the real thing. **Study the concepts** until you understand them fully, and then you'll be able to answer any question that shows up on the test.

It's important to wait on the practice tests until you're ready. If you take a test on your first day of study, you may be overwhelmed by the amount of material covered and how much you need to learn. Work up to it gradually.

On test day, you'll need to be prepared for answering questions, managing your time, and using the test-taking strategies you've learned. It's a lot to balance, like a mental marathon that will have a big impact on your future. Like training for a marathon, you'll need to start slowly and work your way up. When test day arrives, you'll be ready.

Start with the strategies you've read in the first two Secret Keys—plan your course and study in the way that works best for you. If you have time, consider using multiple study resources to get different approaches to the same concepts. It can be helpful to see difficult concepts from more than one angle. Then find a good source for practice tests. Many times, the test website will suggest potential study resources or provide sample tests.

Practice Test Strategy

If you're able to find at least three practice tests, we recommend this strategy:

UNTIMED AND OPEN-BOOK PRACTICE

Take the first test with no time constraints and with your notes and study guide handy. Take your time and focus on applying the strategies you've learned.

TIMED AND OPEN-BOOK PRACTICE

Take the second practice test open-book as well, but set a timer and practice pacing yourself to finish in time.

TIMED AND CLOSED-BOOK PRACTICE

Take any other practice tests as if it were test day. Set a timer and put away your study materials. Sit at a table or desk in a quiet room, imagine yourself at the testing center, and answer questions as quickly and accurately as possible.

Keep repeating timed and closed-book tests on a regular basis until you run out of practice tests or it's time for the actual test. Your mind will be ready for the schedule and stress of test day, and you'll be able to focus on recalling the material you've learned.

Secret Key #4 – Pace Yourself

Once you're fully prepared for the material on the test, your biggest challenge on test day will be managing your time. Just knowing that the clock is ticking can make you panic even if you have plenty of time left. Work on pacing yourself so you can build confidence against the time constraints of the exam. Pacing is a difficult skill to master, especially in a high-pressure environment, so **practice is vital**.

Set time expectations for your pace based on how much time is available. For example, if a section has 60 questions and the time limit is 30 minutes, you know you have to average 30 seconds or less per question in order to answer them all. Although 30 seconds is the hard limit, set 25 seconds per question as your goal, so you reserve extra time to spend on harder questions. When you budget extra time for the harder questions, you no longer have any reason to stress when those questions take longer to answer.

Don't let this time expectation distract you from working through the test at a calm, steady pace, but keep it in mind so you don't spend too much time on any one question. Recognize that taking extra time on one question you don't understand may keep you from answering two that you do understand later in the test. If your time limit for a question is up and you're still not sure of the answer, mark it and move on, and come back to it later if the time and the test format allow. If the testing format doesn't allow you to return to earlier questions, just make an educated guess; then put it out of your mind and move on.

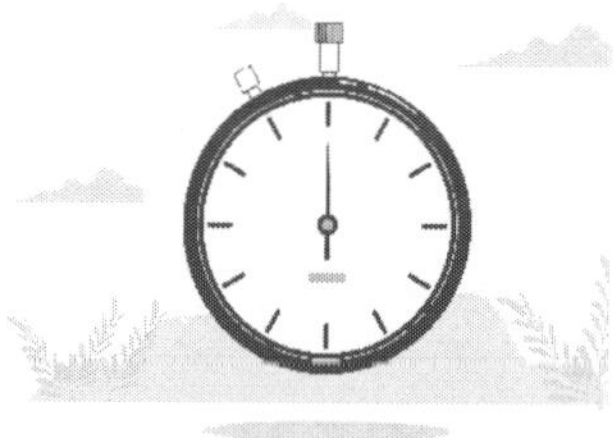

On the easier questions, be careful not to rush. It may seem wise to hurry through them so you have more time for the challenging ones, but it's not worth missing one if you know the concept and just didn't take the time to read the question fully. Work efficiently but make sure you understand the question and have looked at all of the answer choices, since more than one may seem right at first.

Even if you're paying attention to the time, you may find yourself a little behind at some point. You should speed up to get back on track, but do so wisely. Don't panic; just take a few seconds less on each question until you're caught up. Don't guess without thinking, but do look through the answer choices and eliminate any you know are wrong. If you can get down to two choices, it is often worthwhile to guess from those. Once you've chosen an answer, move on and don't dwell on any that you skipped or had to hurry through. If a question was taking too long, chances are it was one of the harder ones, so you weren't as likely to get it right anyway.

On the other hand, if you find yourself getting ahead of schedule, it may be beneficial to slow down a little. The more quickly you work, the more likely you are to make a careless mistake that will affect your score. You've budgeted time for each question, so don't be afraid to spend that time. Practice an efficient but careful pace to get the most out of the time you have.

Secret Key #5 – Have a Plan for Guessing

When you're taking the test, you may find yourself stuck on a question. Some of the answer choices seem better than others, but you don't see the one answer choice that is obviously correct. What do you do?

The scenario described above is very common, yet most test takers have not effectively prepared for it. Developing and practicing a plan for guessing may be one of the single most effective uses of your time as you get ready for the exam.

In developing your plan for guessing, there are three questions to address:

- When should you start the guessing process?
- How should you narrow down the choices?
- Which answer should you choose?

When to Start the Guessing Process

Unless your plan for guessing is to select C every time (which, despite its merits, is not what we recommend), you need to leave yourself enough time to apply your answer elimination strategies. Since you have a limited amount of time for each question, that means that if you're going to give yourself the best shot at guessing correctly, you have to decide quickly whether or not you will guess.

Of course, the best-case scenario is that you don't have to guess at all, so first, see if you can answer the question based on your knowledge of the subject and basic reasoning skills. Focus on the key words in the question and try to jog your memory of related topics. Give yourself a chance to bring the knowledge to mind, but once you realize that you don't have (or you can't access) the knowledge you need to answer the question, it's time to start the guessing process.

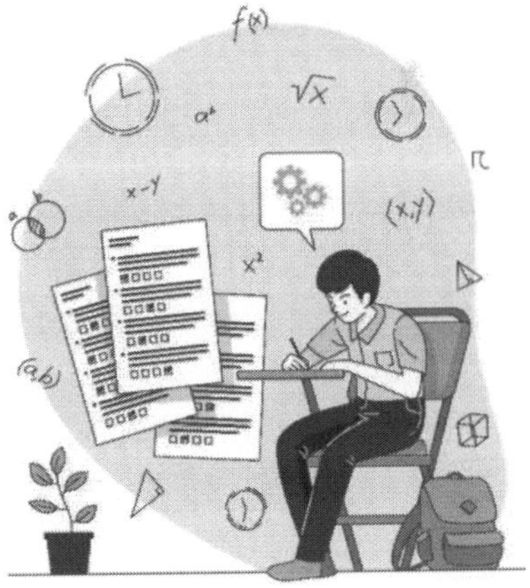

It's almost always better to start the guessing process too early than too late. It only takes a few seconds to remember something and answer the question from knowledge. Carefully eliminating wrong answer choices takes longer. Plus, going through the process of eliminating answer choices can actually help jog your memory.

Summary: Start the guessing process as soon as you decide that you can't answer the question based on your knowledge.

How to Narrow Down the Choices

The next chapter in this book (**Test-Taking Strategies**) includes a wide range of strategies for how to approach questions and how to look for answer choices to eliminate. You will definitely want to read those carefully, practice them, and figure out which ones work best for you. Here though, we're going to address a mindset rather than a particular strategy.

Your odds of guessing an answer correctly depend on how many options you are choosing from.

Number of options left	5	4	3	2	1
Odds of guessing correctly	20%	25%	33%	50%	100%

You can see from this chart just how valuable it is to be able to eliminate incorrect answers and make an educated guess, but there are two things that many test takers do that cause them to miss out on the benefits of guessing:

- Accidentally eliminating the correct answer
- Selecting an answer based on an impression

We'll look at the first one here, and the second one in the next section.

To avoid accidentally eliminating the correct answer, we recommend a thought exercise called **the $5 challenge**. In this challenge, you only eliminate an answer choice from contention if you are willing to bet $5 on it being wrong. Why $5? Five dollars is a small but not insignificant amount of money. It's an amount you could afford to lose but wouldn't want to throw away. And while losing $5 once might not hurt too much, doing it twenty times will set you back $100. In the same way, each small decision you make—eliminating a choice here, guessing on a question there—won't by itself impact your score very much, but when you put them all together, they can make a big difference. By holding each answer choice elimination decision to a higher standard, you can reduce the risk of accidentally eliminating the correct answer.

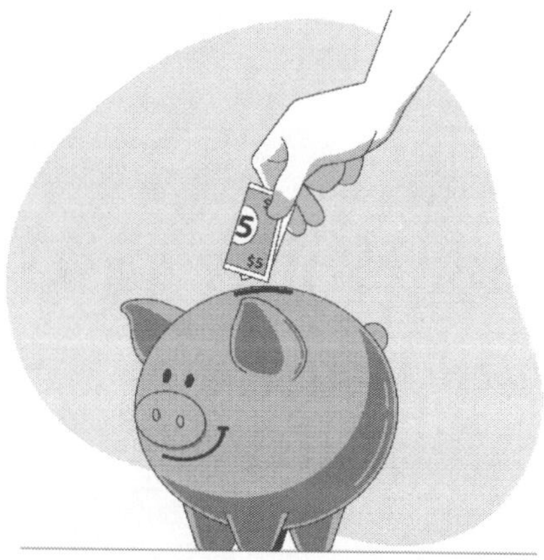

The $5 challenge can also be applied in a positive sense: If you are willing to bet $5 that an answer choice *is* correct, go ahead and mark it as correct.

Summary: Only eliminate an answer choice if you are willing to bet $5 that it is wrong.

Which Answer to Choose

You're taking the test. You've run into a hard question and decided you'll have to guess. You've eliminated all the answer choices you're willing to bet $5 on. Now you have to pick an answer. Why do we even need to talk about this? Why can't you just pick whichever one you feel like when the time comes?

The answer to these questions is that if you don't come into the test with a plan, you'll rely on your impression to select an answer choice, and if you do that, you risk falling into a trap. The test writers know that everyone who takes their test will be guessing on some of the questions, so they intentionally write wrong answer choices to seem plausible. You still have to pick an answer though, and if the wrong answer choices are designed to look right, how can you ever be sure that you're not falling for their trap? The best solution we've found to this dilemma is to take the decision out of your hands entirely. Here is the process we recommend:

Once you've eliminated any choices that you are confident (willing to bet $5) are wrong, select the first remaining choice as your answer.

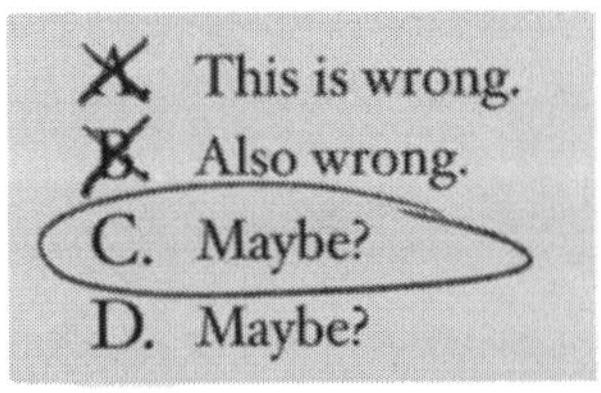

Whether you choose to select the first remaining choice, the second, or the last, the important thing is that you use some preselected standard. Using this approach guarantees that you will not be enticed into selecting an answer choice that looks right, because you are not basing your decision on how the answer choices look.

This is not meant to make you question your knowledge. Instead, it is to help you recognize the difference between your knowledge and your impressions. There's a huge difference between thinking an answer is right because of what you know, and thinking an answer is right because it looks or sounds like it should be right.

Summary: To ensure that your selection is appropriately random, make a predetermined selection from among all answer choices you have not eliminated.

Test-Taking Strategies

This section contains a list of test-taking strategies that you may find helpful as you work through the test. By taking what you know and applying logical thought, you can maximize your chances of answering any question correctly!

It is very important to realize that every question is different and every person is different: no single strategy will work on every question, and no single strategy will work for every person. That's why we've included all of them here, so you can try them out and determine which ones work best for different types of questions and which ones work best for you.

Question Strategies

✓ Read Carefully

Read the question and the answer choices carefully. Don't miss the question because you misread the terms. You have plenty of time to read each question thoroughly and make sure you understand what is being asked. Yet a happy medium must be attained, so don't waste too much time. You must read carefully and efficiently.

✓ Contextual Clues

Look for contextual clues. If the question includes a word you are not familiar with, look at the immediate context for some indication of what the word might mean. Contextual clues can often give you all the information you need to decipher the meaning of an unfamiliar word. Even if you can't determine the meaning, you may be able to narrow down the possibilities enough to make a solid guess at the answer to the question.

✓ Prefixes

If you're having trouble with a word in the question or answer choices, try dissecting it. Take advantage of every clue that the word might include. Prefixes can be a huge help. Usually, they allow you to determine a basic meaning. *Pre-* means before, *post-* means after, *pro-* is positive, *de-* is negative. From prefixes, you can get an idea of the general meaning of the word and try to put it into context.

✓ Hedge Words

Watch out for critical hedge words, such as *likely, may, can, often, almost, mostly, usually, generally, rarely,* and *sometimes.* Question writers insert these hedge phrases to cover every possibility. Often an answer choice will be wrong simply because it leaves no room for exception. Be on guard for answer choices that have definitive words such as *exactly* and *always.*

✓ Switchback Words

Stay alert for *switchbacks.* These are the words and phrases frequently used to alert you to shifts in thought. The most common switchback words are *but, although,* and *however.* Others include *nevertheless, on the other hand, even though, while, in spite of, despite,* and *regardless of.* Switchback words are important to catch because they can change the direction of the question or an answer choice.

✓ Face Value

When in doubt, use common sense. Accept the situation in the problem at face value. Don't read too much into it. These problems will not require you to make wild assumptions. If you have to go beyond creativity and warp time or space in order to have an answer choice fit the question, then you should move on and consider the other answer choices. These are normal problems rooted in reality. The applicable relationship or explanation may not be readily apparent, but it is there for you to figure out. Use your common sense to interpret anything that isn't clear.

Answer Choice Strategies

ANSWER SELECTION

The most thorough way to pick an answer choice is to identify and eliminate wrong answers until only one is left, then confirm it is the correct answer. Sometimes an answer choice may immediately seem right, but be careful. The test writers will usually put more than one reasonable answer choice on each question, so take a second to read all of them and make sure that the other choices are not equally obvious. As long as you have time left, it is better to read every answer choice than to pick the first one that looks right without checking the others.

ANSWER CHOICE FAMILIES

An answer choice family consists of two (in rare cases, three) answer choices that are very similar in construction and cannot all be true at the same time. If you see two answer choices that are direct opposites or parallels, one of them is usually the correct answer. For instance, if one answer choice says that quantity *x* increases and another either says that quantity *x* decreases (opposite) or says that quantity *y* increases (parallel), then those answer choices would fall into the same family. An answer choice that doesn't match the construction of the answer choice family is more likely to be incorrect. Most questions will not have answer choice families, but when they do appear, you should be prepared to recognize them.

ELIMINATE ANSWERS

Eliminate answer choices as soon as you realize they are wrong, but make sure you consider all possibilities. If you are eliminating answer choices and realize that the last one you are left with is also wrong, don't panic. Start over and consider each choice again. There may be something you missed the first time that you will realize on the second pass.

AVOID FACT TRAPS

Don't be distracted by an answer choice that is factually true but doesn't answer the question. You are looking for the choice that answers the question. Stay focused on what the question is asking for so you don't accidentally pick an answer that is true but incorrect. Always go back to the question and make sure the answer choice you've selected actually answers the question and is not merely a true statement.

EXTREME STATEMENTS

In general, you should avoid answers that put forth extreme actions as standard practice or proclaim controversial ideas as established fact. An answer choice that states the "process should be used in certain situations, if..." is much more likely to be correct than one that states the "process should be discontinued completely." The first is a calm rational statement and doesn't even make a definitive, uncompromising stance, using a hedge word *if* to provide wiggle room, whereas the second choice is far more extreme.

BENCHMARK

As you read through the answer choices and you come across one that seems to answer the question well, mentally select that answer choice. This is not your final answer, but it's the one that will help you evaluate the other answer choices. The one that you selected is your benchmark or standard for judging each of the other answer choices. Every other answer choice must be compared to your benchmark. That choice is correct until proven otherwise by another answer choice beating it. If you find a better answer, then that one becomes your new benchmark. Once you've decided that no other choice answers the question as well as your benchmark, you have your final answer.

⊘ PREDICT THE ANSWER

Before you even start looking at the answer choices, it is often best to try to predict the answer. When you come up with the answer on your own, it is easier to avoid distractions and traps because you will know exactly what to look for. The right answer choice is unlikely to be word-for-word what you came up with, but it should be a close match. Even if you are confident that you have the right answer, you should still take the time to read each option before moving on.

General Strategies

⊘ TOUGH QUESTIONS

If you are stumped on a problem or it appears too hard or too difficult, don't waste time. Move on! Remember though, if you can quickly check for obviously incorrect answer choices, your chances of guessing correctly are greatly improved. Before you completely give up, at least try to knock out a couple of possible answers. Eliminate what you can and then guess at the remaining answer choices before moving on.

⊘ CHECK YOUR WORK

Since you will probably not know every term listed and the answer to every question, it is important that you get credit for the ones that you do know. Don't miss any questions through careless mistakes. If at all possible, try to take a second to look back over your answer selection and make sure you've selected the correct answer choice and haven't made a costly careless mistake (such as marking an answer choice that you didn't mean to mark). This quick double check should more than pay for itself in caught mistakes for the time it costs.

⊘ PACE YOURSELF

It's easy to be overwhelmed when you're looking at a page full of questions; your mind is confused and full of random thoughts, and the clock is ticking down faster than you would like. Calm down and maintain the pace that you have set for yourself. Especially as you get down to the last few minutes of the test, don't let the small numbers on the clock make you panic. As long as you are on track by monitoring your pace, you are guaranteed to have time for each question.

⊘ DON'T RUSH

It is very easy to make errors when you are in a hurry. Maintaining a fast pace in answering questions is pointless if it makes you miss questions that you would have gotten right otherwise. Test writers like to include distracting information and wrong answers that seem right. Taking a little extra time to avoid careless mistakes can make all the difference in your test score. Find a pace that allows you to be confident in the answers that you select.

⊘ KEEP MOVING

Panicking will not help you pass the test, so do your best to stay calm and keep moving. Taking deep breaths and going through the answer elimination steps you practiced can help to break through a stress barrier and keep your pace.

Final Notes

The combination of a solid foundation of content knowledge and the confidence that comes from practicing your plan for applying that knowledge is the key to maximizing your performance on test day. As your foundation of content knowledge is built up and strengthened, you'll find that the strategies included in this chapter become more and more effective in helping you quickly sift through the distractions and traps of the test to isolate the correct answer.

Now that you're preparing to move forward into the test content chapters of this book, be sure to keep your goal in mind. As you read, think about how you will be able to apply this information on the test. If you've already seen sample questions for the test and you have an idea of the question format and style, try to come up with questions of your own that you can answer based on what you're reading. This will give you valuable practice applying your knowledge in the same ways you can expect to on test day.

Good luck and good studying!

Assessment

Patient Interviews

Interview Process and Techniques

The care provider should review previous medical records, have a clear idea of the purpose of the interview, and outline the questions. If possible, the patient should be interviewed alone or should be asked if he or she wants family members present. Both verbal and nonverbal responses should be observed during an interview. Important factors include:

- **Initial introductions**: Make introductions by name and explain roles and the purpose of the interview, asking how the patient wishes to be addressed and avoiding using familiar terms, such as "dear," which may be considered condescending. Stress the confidential nature of the interview and explain who will receive the information.
- **Interview structure**: The interview may be somewhat unstructured, guided by patient responses, or may be very structured with the care provider asking a list of questions, but he or she must remain flexible while still guiding the discussion in order to accommodate different communication styles.
- **Appearance**: The care provider should be professionally dressed and wearing a clear nametag. The patient's appearance should be observed non-judgmentally for clothes (loose/tight clothes may indicate weight change), cleanliness (dirty clothes/skin/hair may indicate cognitive or physical impairment or poverty), and demeanor (calm, fidgeting, nervous).

History Collection During Initial Patient Interview

In order to plan for optimal wound management, history collection during the initial patient interview should include as much information about the wound as possible. Information should include:

- Type of wound, size, and location
- Etiology of the wound (known, unknown)
- Duration of wound
- Degree of pain associated with the wound (increasing, decreasing)
- All previous treatments/interventions (both medical and patient-initiated), including types of dressings
- Changes in the wound (increase in size, decrease in size, tunneling, wound edges, and wound color)
- Evidence of necrosis, exudate, edema, granulation tissue, epithelial tissue, induration, erythema, and cyanosis
- Presence of odor (character of odor and amount of exudate)
- Nutritional status, including fluid intake, supplements, vitamins, and usual diet
- Medical history, including diseases, injuries, surgeries, and hospitalizations
- Lifestyle, including homelessness
- Habits, including use of tobacco, alcohol, and illicit substances
- List of medications, including OTC, traditional medicines (such as herbs), and prescribed medications
- Recent laboratory work (CBC, FBS, A1c)
- Mobility issues

Issues of Cultural Diversity During the Interview and Assessment

Issues of cultural diversity must be considered during the initial interview and the wound assessment. Individuals vary considerably in their attitudes, so assuming that all members of an ethnic or cultural group share the same values is never valid. The individual must be assessed as well as the group. It is important to take time to observe family dynamics and language barriers, arranging for translators if necessary to ensure that there is adequate communication. In patriarchal cultures, such as the Mexican culture, the eldest male may speak for the patient. In some Muslim cultures, females will resist care by males. Acknowledging biological differences, such as skin color, is important for assessing skin because wounds and bruising may have a different appearance. The attitudes and beliefs of the patient in relation to wound care must be understood, accepted, and treated with respect. In some cases, the use of healers or cultural traditions must be incorporated into a plan of care.

Anatomy and Physiology of the Skins

Epidermis

The epidermis is the outer avascular layer of skin. It is composed of stratified squamous epithelial cells (keratinocytes) and regenerates every 4-6 weeks. Layers of the epidermis consist of the following:

- **Stratum corneum**, the outer layer, is flattened dead keratinized cells (corneocytes), providing a waterproof barrier against microorganisms and injury.
- **Stratum lucidum** is 1-5 translucent cells thick and is found in the palms and soles of the feet where the skin is thicker.
- **Stratum granulosum** is 1-5 cells thick and contains keratinocytes with granules that contain proteins.
- **Stratum spinosum** (prickly layers) contains spiny desmosomes that join cube-like cells in multiple layers, providing structure and support.
- **Stratum germinativum/stratum basale** is one layer of active undifferentiated basal cells with a basement membrane zone beneath.

Cells ascend into the stratum spinosum and become keratinocytes. It can take 2-3 weeks for a cell to leave the basal layer and move upward to the stratum corneum, replenishing the various layers. The basal layer contains melanocytes, which provide pigmentation and protection from sunlight.

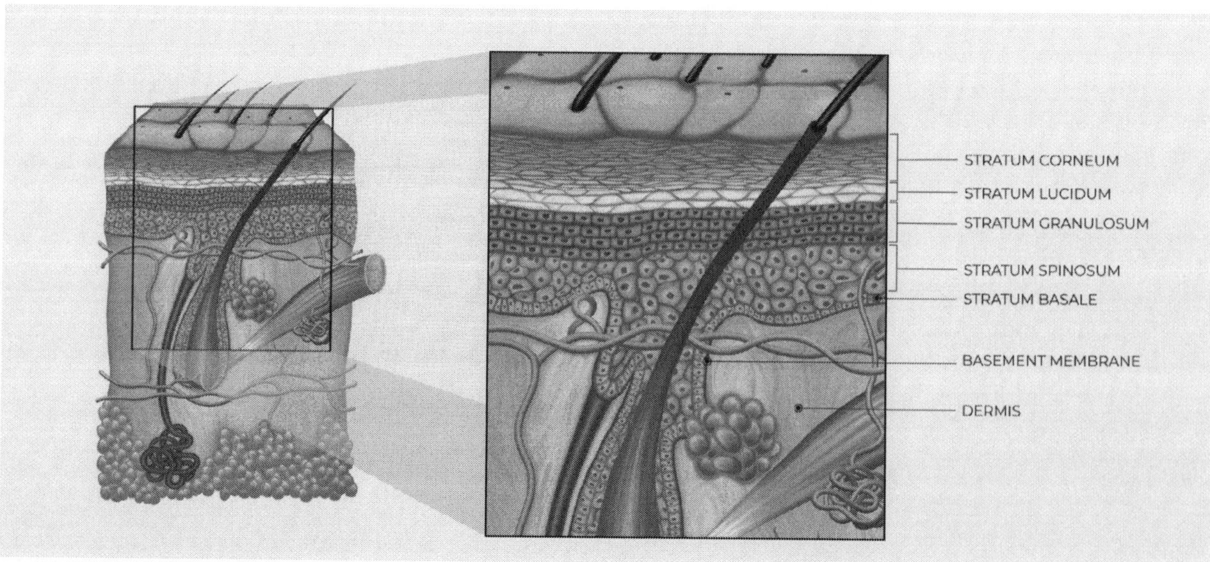

Basement Membrane Zone

The junction of the epidermis and dermis is the **basement membrane zone** (BMZ), which provides support for the cells above. It comprises two layers:

- **Lamina lucida** (because of translucent electrons) contains glycoprotein laminin.
- **Lamina densa** (because of dense electrons) comprises type IV collagen.

Lamina reticularis (bottom portion) is synthesized by cells in connective tissues beneath and contains fibronectin. It contains Type I, II, III and sometimes IV collagen. It serves as the interface between the basement membrane and the underlying connective tissue.

The anchoring structures are composed of hemidesmosomes, which the basal keratocytes use with anchoring filaments and fibrils to attach. BMZ antibodies have been found that react to various antigens. Langerhans cells are part of the immune system. The BMZ is affected by blister formation and disrupted during healing of wounds. The BMZ is modified in skin with psoriasis, affecting adhesion, migration, proliferation, and differentiation of keratinocytes, interfering with the normal function of the basement membrane.

Dermis and Hypodermis

The dermis is the layer beneath the epidermis and BMZ. The dermis contains nerves, sebaceous glands, sweat glands, hair follicles, lymphatic vessels, veins, and arteries. Fibroblasts produce the primary proteins of this layer, collagen and elastin, with a protein substance called **ground substance** in the space between them. Mast cells, macrophages, and lymphocytes, which are all involved in the skin immune system (SIS), are also found in the dermis. There are **two areas of the dermis**:

- **Papillary dermis** contains the vascular networks that support the epidermis with oxygen and nutrients. It also functions in thermoregulation by regulating blood flow and contains sensory nerve endings.
- **Reticular dermis** contains the hair follicles and glands and is comprised of connective tissue with collagen and elastic fibers that provides elasticity and strength to the skin. It also contains blood vessels.

The **hypodermis** comprises the layer of subcutaneous tissue below the dermis, providing vasculature, cushioning, and insulation.

Functions of the Skin

The primary functions of the skin are the following:

- **Protection**: The skin provides a waterproof barrier to protect against microorganisms, chemicals, and ultraviolet radiation through pigmentation provided by melanocytes.
- **Immunity**: The skin immune system (SIS) with the Langerhans cells protects against foreign antigens. Mast cells and macrophages destroy pathogenic microorganisms as well as promote tissue repair and wound healing.
- **Sensation**: The nerve endings are found in the skin, allowing the person to sense pain, pressure, and temperature. Combinations of sensations detected by nerve receptors translate into sensations of burning, itching, and tickling.
- **Thermoregulation**: The blood vessels within the skin help control body temperature by constricting to retain body heat, or dilating to release heat.
- **Metabolism**: Ultraviolet radiation converts 7-dehydrocholesteral to cholecalciferol, Vitamin D. Vitamin D is synthesized within the skin and then transmits to other parts of the body. It is critical in the metabolism of calcium and phosphate for the formation of bone.
- **Appearance**: Skin provides a cosmetic appearance and communicates identification.

Review Video: Integumentary System
Visit mometrix.com/academy and enter code: 655980

Musculoskeletal System and the Skin

The musculoskeletal system includes 203 bones: long bones (femur), short bones (carpal), and flat bones (sternum). The outer hard shell of the bone is the cortex and the inner porous area is the trabecular bone. The skeletal system is connected by tendons and cartilage and protected, supported, and allowed movement by about 700 soft tissue muscles. Muscles are comprised of muscle fibers. Muscle tissue is contractile and elastic and allows movement of body parts by shortening and lengthening. There are three types of muscles in the human body:

- **Skeletal muscle**: Voluntary muscles that are attached to bones of the head, neck, arms, and legs and facilitate movement
- **Smooth muscle**: Involuntary muscles that make up the walls of blood vessels and hollow organs, such as the bladder
- **Cardiac muscle**: Involuntary muscles comprised of muscle cells found only in the heart

While the skeletal system provides support, it also increases the risk of pressure sores and delays healing when tissue is compressed between bone and surface. The muscles have a high demand for oxygen and are fed by many blood vessels, which are also critical for wound healing. When wounds damage muscles, the blood flow may be interrupted.

Vascular System and the Skin

The vascular system comprises the venous system and the arterial system. The venous system includes veins, venules, and venous capillaries. Deoxygenated venous blood returns to the heart per the inferior vena cava, superior vena cava, and coronary sinus (bringing blood from the coronary arteries) into the right atrium, then through the tricuspid valve to the right ventricle and through the pulmonic valve into the lungs to exchange carbon dioxide for oxygen. The oxygenated blood returns through the pulmonary veins to the left atrium, through the mitral valve, into the left ventricle, through the aortic valve, and into the aorta and arterial system. The arterial system includes the coronary arteries (which branch from the aorta after it leaves the heart) and arteries, arterioles, and arterial capillaries. In response to a wound, vasoconstriction occurs to reduce bleeding, and clots form to close the wound. This is followed by vasodilation to provide nutrients to the wound and phagocytosis to fight infection and provide growth factors. Angiogenesis increases circulation to healing tissue.

Review Video: Cardiovascular System
Visit mometrix.com/academy and enter code: 376581

Neurological System and the Skin

The neurological (nervous) system consists of the central nervous system (CNS) (brain, spinal cord and nerves) and the peripheral nervous system (PNS) (sensory neurons, ganglia [nerve clusters], and nerves connecting to the central nervous system). The brain consists of the cerebrum (frontal, temporal, parietal, and occipital lobes) the cerebellum, and the brainstem, which is continuous with the spinal cord. The PNS is divided into the autonomic nervous system and the somatic nervous system. The autonomic nervous system, which comprises the parasympathetic and sympathetic nervous systems, controls the body's organs and maintains homeostasis (balance). The SNS plays an important role in angiogenesis, which is critical to wound healing. Functions of the autonomic nervous system include heart rate and function, respiration, digestion, sexual arousal, and other systems. The somatic nervous system comprises cranial and spinal nerves that connect the central nervous system to the skeletal muscles and skin. The somatic nervous system is the voluntarily-controlled component of the peripheral nervous system, and it receives and responds to external sensory stimuli from the skin (such as from pressure or wound pain) and sensory organs.

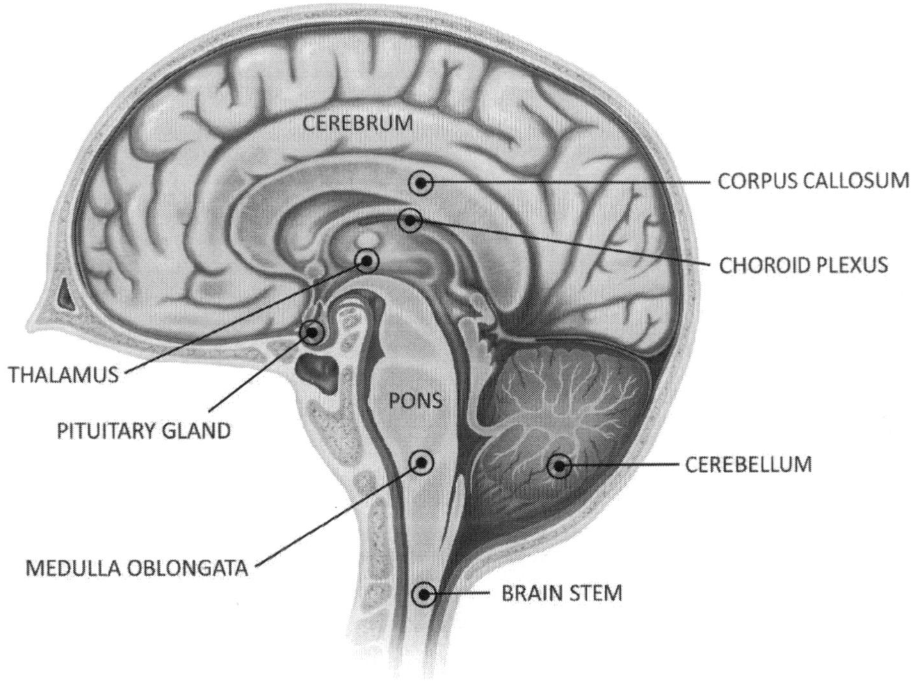

Lymphatic System and the Skin

The lymphatic system absorbs fluids (lymph) from the blood into the interstitial spaces, carries excess fluids back to the bloodstream, absorbs fatty acids from the intestines, and transports them to the blood. The lymphatic system can also transport cancerous cells from one organ to another. The lymphatic system includes the thymus gland, the spleen, lymph nodes, bone marrow, and lymphatic pathways. The **thymus gland** contains lymphocytes and secretes thymosins, which stimulate maturation of T lymphocytes, a critical cell necessary to fight infections. The **spleen** serves as a reservoir of blood, filters blood, promotes phagocytosis, provides antibodies to strip capsules from bacteria, and produces blood cells if bone marrow not functioning properly). **Lymph nodes** filter harmful particles and provide immune surveillance and are primarily in the cervical, axillary, supratrochlear, thoracic, abdominal, pelvic, and inguinal areas. **Bone marrow** produces blood cells and **lymphatic pathways** (vessels, capillaries, trunks, collecting ducts) carry the lymph through the body. As part of wound healing, lymphatic vessels must regenerate. Lymphatic dysfunction with edema can impair circulation, delay healing, promote bacterial colonization, and result in fibrosis of tissue and chronic inflammation.

Wound Healing

PRIMARY, SECONDARY, AND TERTIARY HEALING

Primary healing (healing by first intention) involves a wound that is surgically closed by suturing, flaps, or split or full-thickness grafts to completely cover the wound. Primary healing is the most common approach used for surgeries or repair of wounds or lacerations, especially when the wound is essentially "clean."

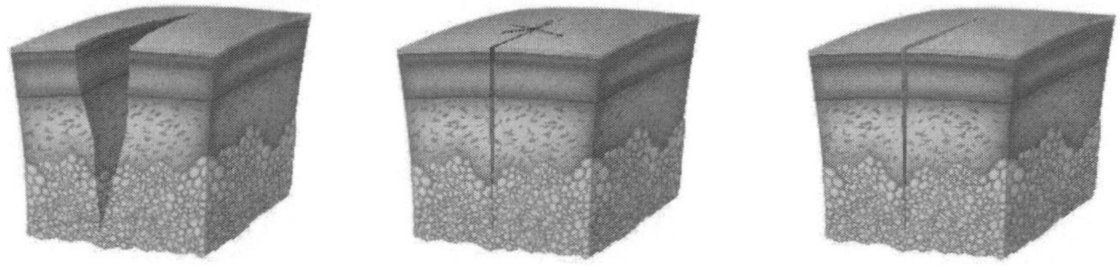

Secondary healing (healing by second intention) involves leaving the wound open and allowing it to close through granulation and epithelialization. Debridement of the wound is done to prepare the wound bed for healing. This approach may be used with contaminated "dirty" or infected wounds to prevent abscess formation and allow the wound to drain.

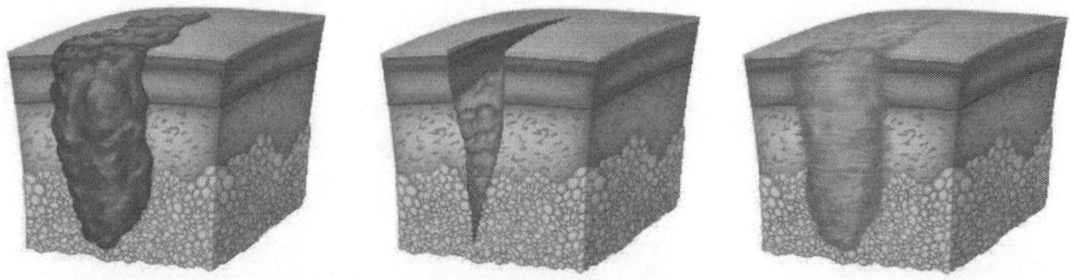

Tertiary healing (healing by third intention) is also sometimes called delayed primary closure because it involves first debriding the wound and allowing it to begin healing while open and then later closing the wound through suturing or grafts. This approach is common with wounds that are contaminated, such as severe animal bites, or wounds related to mixed trauma.

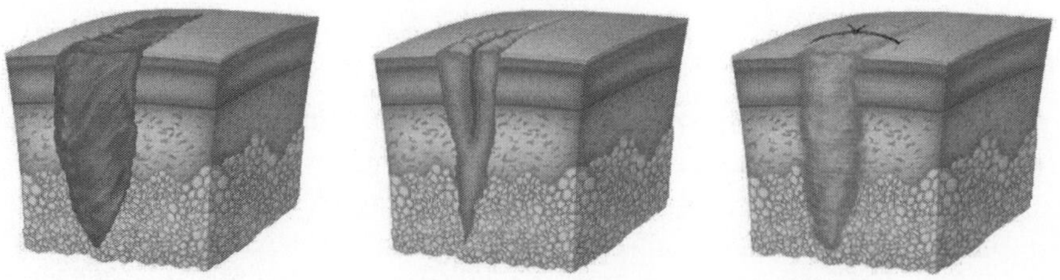

Phases of Wound Healing

There are **four phases of wound healing**:

1. **Hemostasis** is the first phase of wound healing, occurring within minutes of injury. After the wound occurs, the blood vessels constrict to decrease bleeding. Platelets gather to form a clot and then secrete factors, which cause the production of thrombin. This stimulates fibrin formation from fibrinogen. The resultant clot is a strong one, which becomes the serosanguinous crust (scab) for the wound. Platelets secrete cytokines, including platelet-derived growth factor that begins the healing process.
2. The **inflammation phase** occurs next and lasts about four days normally. Blood vessels in the area leak plasma and neutrophils into the wound, causing erythema, edema, and increased warmth. Any debris or microorganisms are destroyed by the neutrophils and localized mast cells through phagocytosis. When fibrin is broken down, it attracts macrophages to the area. They also destroy microorganisms and secrete growth factors to stimulate the next phase of healing.
3. The **proliferative phase** occurs over about days 5-20 in normal healing. During the proliferative phase, fibroblasts secrete collagen to manufacture a framework within the wound. New capillaries sprout from damaged vessel ends in a process called angiogenesis. Keratinocytes cause epithelialization in which new skin cells form at the edges of the wound, migrating inward to meet in the center of the defect. Approximately five days after a wound occurs, the fibroblasts and myofibroblasts contract to bring the wound edges closer, resulting in a smaller defect.
4. **Remodeling or maturation** of a wound begins about 21 days after the wound occurs and continues over the next year. Collagen is deposited, eventually resulting in a stiff, strong scar that has 70-80% of the tensile strength of normal skin. Blood vessels in the newly formed tissues gradually disappear from the scar during this phase.

Wound Healing on the Cellular Level

Cytokines are proteins that serve as soluble mediators and are essential to wound healing. They include growth factors, tumor necrosis factors, interferons, and interleukins. Cytokines are produced from platelets, fibroblasts, monocytes, endothelial cells, and macrophages and facilitate communication between cells and regulate cell proliferation and inflammatory reactions as part of healing. Cytokines also attract neutrophils and macrophages. Cells in the wound produce extracellular matrix proteins. The extracellular matrix includes fibrous and adhesive proteins (collagen, elastin, laminin, fibronectin) and polysaccharides (proteoglycans and glycosaminoglycans [GAGs]). Following injury, platelets aggregate and degranulate, activating factor XII (Hagerman), which promotes formation of a fibrinous clot, which then activates fibrinolysis to break down the clot triggering the complement system. Platelet degranulation triggers release of cytokines into the wound, including:

- **Platelet-derived growth factor (PDGF)**: Activates immune cells and fibroblasts, promotes formation of extracellular matrix and angiogenesis.
- **Fibroblast growth factor (FGF) and epidermal growth factor (EGF)**: Increases proliferation/migration of keratinocytes and extracellular matrix deposition, epithelial cell proliferation, angiogenesis, and formation of granulation tissue.
- **Transforming growth factor (TGFα and TGFβ)**: Promotes formation of extracellular matrix, reduces scarring, increases collagen and tissue inhibitors of metalloproteinase synthesis, decreasing collagen and fibronectin.
- **Tumor necrosis factor α**: Expressed by macrophages to stimulate angiogenesis.

Partial-Thickness and Full-Thickness Wound Healing

Partial-thickness wounds involve only the epidermis and the upper parts of the dermis, so the underlying structures that repair skin and provide nutrients, such as the vasculature, and protection, such as the glands, remain intact. Bleeding activates hemostasis and provides a temporary bacterial barrier. Coagulation occurs and fibrin is formed with the clot sealing disrupted vessels. This is followed by fibrinolysis, during which the clot breaks down and repair begins with the inflammatory stage. Healing phase's progress and wounds usually heal within about 2 weeks.

Full-thickness wounds involve the loss of the epidermis and dermis and may also involve loss of underlying tissues, through the fascia, muscle, and to the bone. Full-thickness wounds may be acute or chronic and heal by primary or secondary intention. Those healing by secondary intention are usually surgical wounds that have dehisced or those resulting from underlying morbidities that interfere with normal healing. Bleeding and hemostasis do not occur with healing by secondary intention, compromising the healing process.

Acute and Chronic Wound Healing

Acute wounds are usually related to an injury and bleed freely because circulation is unimpaired. They heal quickly and continuously, going through the phases of healing in a predictable manner for the size of the wound. There are few if any complications in the healing process.

Chronic wounds are associated with problems in healing, often because of underlying arterial insufficiency. There may not be normal functioning of the components in the healing process or the components may be delayed. For example, the inflammatory phase of healing is usually prolonged. Normal regulatory signals that cause growth to occur may be ignored by the body. There may be repeated injuries to the area, increased inflammation, and poor supply of oxygen and nutrients to the wound. There may be host factors, such as smoking and malnutrition that hamper healing. Genetic and systemic disease can both result in chronic wounds that fail to heal.

Microenvironmental Factors That Affect Wound Healing

Wound microenvironment refers to the condition of the wound bed. One problem is that there is often insufficient bleeding in the wound microenvironment initially, so there is less thrombin produced and this impairs production of fibrin. There may be an inadequate supply of growth factors. The lack of growth factors prevents the proliferation of new cells. Lack of innervation may further impair healing. The inflammatory phase is often prolonged, and there is inadequate debridement as phagocytosis is impaired. The presence of infection competes with newly forming skin cells for adequate oxygen and nutrients. The toxins from bacteria further pollute the microenvironment. Moisture is necessary for repair but the presence of excess exudate can restrict cell growth and introduce harmful proteases that further break down growth factors.

Signs of Wound Healing

The wound bed must be examined to determine the color of the tissues, amount of moisture present, and degree of epithelialization to demonstrate **signs of healing**:

- Granulation tissue has a granular appearance, is beefy red, feels soft and sponge-like to the touch, bleeds readily when probed, and exhibits no twitch when pinched. It must be distinguished from non-granular tissue, which is smooth and red, and not healing, and hypergranulation, which is soft and spongy and rises above the level of the wound and interferes with epithelialization.
- Epithelialization migrates out from the edges of the wound towards the center. Tissue is usually dry and appears light pink or violet-colored.

The wound bed may show a combination of slough, necrotic tissue, and granular tissue at the same time, so the percentage of each should be determined so that the progress of epithelialization can be demonstrated over time. Pain should be assessed as it may indicate infection.

Scarring

Factors Influencing the Amount of Scar Tissue Formed

Deeper wounds produce more scar tissue because a larger amount of granulation tissue is deposited over a longer period of time. The amount of inflammation in a wound also helps to determine the amount of scar tissue formed. Highly pigmented skin produces more scar tissue as does a genetic propensity towards scarring.

Tension on a wound during healing causes tissue damage and increased inflammation. This tension is increased in the young versus an older person due to tighter skin and more activity, so children form larger scars than elderly people. Wound location also contributes to scar formation.

Excessive Scarring

Excessive scarring includes hypertrophic and keloid scars, which are characterized by raised scars that are erythematous and itchy. Excessive scarring is more common in darkly pigmented skin or in areas where the tissue may stretch, such as over joints. Young or pregnant patients or those with a family history of excessive scarring are at increased risk. There are some distinctions between hypertrophic and keloid scars:

- **Hypertrophic scars** most frequently occur over joints where there is tension on the wound (dorsum of the feet, buttocks, shoulder and upper arms, and upper back). They remain localized to the area of the original wound and may spontaneously regress. Scars that form over joints can cause limited mobility as they contract and may need surgical revision to allow more normal movement.
- **Keloid scars** most frequently occur on the upper back and chest as well as the deltoids and earlobes. They extend beyond the original wound and rarely regress. They usually arise after the wound has healed as raised, shiny, rope-like fibrous scars. They do not result in contracture of the wound. Keloids are most common in those with darker skin and occur due to excess collagen deposition, causing increased growth.

Scarless Healing

Scarless healing occurs in the early-gestation fetus, during the first 2 trimesters, but this ability to heal without scars is lost during the 3rd trimester. This is important for intrauterine surgical procedures, commonly performed during the second trimester when abnormalities become evident. The fetus heals without scarring for a variety of reasons:

- Platelet aggregation is lessened, resulting in less growth factor, such as PDGF.
- The inflammatory response is lessened because of immaturity of the immune system and lack of inflammatory cytokines.
- Wounds move quickly from the inflammatory to the proliferative stage of healing. Fibroblasts, keratinocytes, and endothelial cells, critical to tissue formation, rapidly cover the wound bed. There is no contraction or scarring of the wound.
- Growth factors are balanced so they stimulate growth of connective tissue but prevent excess from forming.
- New and native collagen is indistinguishable, so the new tissue remains flexible.

Non-Healing Wounds

Characteristics of non-healing wounds include:

- **Infection**: Infection increases pro-inflammatory cytokines and prolongs the inflammatory phase of wound healing, sometimes resulting in a non-healing chronic wound. Growth factors may degrade. With infection, granulation tissue may appear dusky. Common pathogens include *Staphylococcus aureus, Pseudomonas aeruginosa,* and β-hemolytic *streptococci.*
- **Biofilm**: A dense thin layer of bacteria in a moist adhesive matrix of secreted polymers that clings to the surface of wounds. Multiple bacteria may be present in a biofilm. The biofilm is resistant to antibiotics and to phagocytosis by white blood cells, resulting in degrading and/or non-healing wounds. Biofilms on the surface of wounds may be mechanically removed.
- **Closed edge**: The wound edges become rolled/curled, dry, and hyperkeratotic and fail to advance, a condition referred to as epibole. Epibole appear light-colored in comparison to surrounding tissue, rounded, and firm. Causes include impaired wound bed, infection, hypoxia, drying, and trauma.

Factors That Affect Skin's Ability to Heal

Age

Age is an important consideration when evaluating the skin because the characteristics of the skin change as people age.

- An **infant's** skin is thinner than an adult's because, while the epidermis is developed, the dermis layer is only about 60% of that of an adult and continues to develop after birth. The skin of premature infants is especially friable, allowing for transepidermal water loss and evaporative heat loss.
- During **adolescence**, the hair follicles activate, the thickness of the dermis decreases about 20%, and epidermal turnover time increases, so healing slows.
- As people **continue to age**, Langerhans' cells decrease in number, making the skin more prone to cancer, and the inflammatory reactions decrease. The sweat glands, vascularity, and subcutaneous fat all decrease, interfering with thermoregulation and contributing to dryness and irritation of the skin. The epidermal-dermal junction flattens, resulting in skin that is prone to tearing. The elastin in the skin degrades with age and solar exposure. The thinning of the hypodermis can lead to pressure injuries.

Review Video: Integumentary System
Visit mometrix.com/academy and enter code: 655980

Lotions, Oils, and Soaps

Lotions, oils, and soaps all have an effect on the skin. Many oils and lotions are used to increase hydration of the skin. These can include oil baths, which have a minimal effect on hydration but do increase the skin-surface lipids. Lipids are the fatty substances that surround skin cells, and those in the outer layer of skin, the stratum corneum, with fatty acids form the water barrier to retain skin hydration and soften skin. Sebum, produced by the sebaceous glands, is also a lipid. Applying lotion increases the hydration of the epidermis, giving the skin a smoother appearance, and moisturizing lotions also increase the lipids, providing some protection. Alkaline soaps, on the other hand, removes the lipid coating of the skin for about 45 minutes after a normal washing and may increase dryness and susceptibility to bacterial infection. Alcohol and acetone also remove the lipid coating and can increase dehydration of the skin. Acidic cleaners are less irritating than either neutral or alkaline cleaners.

Sun Exposure

Sun exposure is one of the primary factors in aging of the skin, referred to as photoaging or dermatoheliosis. Tanning occurs when ultraviolet radiation (UVR) damages the epidermis and stimulates the production of melanin as a protective mechanism to prevent damage to deeper layers of skin. When the melanin is overpowered, sunburn results, damaging the outer layers of the skin and sometimes the DNA of the skin cells, which can lead to cancer. There are several effects of photoaging that should be noted in assessment:

- Decrease in elasticity and strength
- Dry, rough, wrinkled skin
- Fine veins on face and ears
- Freckles and large brown macules (solar lentigines, liver spots) on face, and exposed areas, such as hands and arms and white macules on exposed areas of upper and lower extremities
- Benign lesions, such as actinic and seborrheic keratoses
- Malignant lesions, such as basal cell and squamous cell carcinoma

MEDICATIONS

Medications are a frequent cause of dermatologic effects that can impair the integrity of the skin:

- **Photosensitivity** can be either photoallergic with exposure to ultraviolet radiation causing an allergic reaction, usually with rash, erythema, edema, and pruritus or phototoxic with the drug being converted into a toxin that causes edema, pain, and pronounced erythema. Thiazide diuretics and conjugated estrogens often cause photosensitive reactions.
- **Allergic reactions** may involve rash, urticaria or more complex reactions, such as serum sickness. Amoxicillin alone or with clavulanate causes a high rate of these reactions.
- **Erythema multiforme** has been caused by nifedipine, verapamil, and diltiazem (calcium channel blockers).
- **Toxic epidermal necrolysis** with full-thickness loss of epidermis can be caused by ciprofloxacin.
- **Thinning or atrophy of the skin** because of a loss of collagen and telangiectasia (spider veins) are associated with oral, topical, and inhaled corticosteroids.

LOCAL FACTORS

Local factors that may impact the healing process include:

- **Local infection**: Invasion of the wound by microorganisms, such as *Staphylococcus aureus, MRSA, Pseudomonas,* and *Escherichia coli,* not only slows healing but may cause the wound to erode and increase in size, increasing the risk of systemic infection. Inflammation is a normal part of the healing process, but prolonged inflammation delays healing.
- **Repeat trauma**: If a wound is not adequately protected or if the patient is not positioned correctly, further erosion of the wound may occur.
- **Impaired tissue oxygenation**: Conditions that result in vasoconstriction or low blood flow to the area (such as PAD, blood clot, and hypotension) of the wound can impair healing or worsen the wound. Wounds are typically hypoxic initially because of disruption of blood flow and increased need for oxygen, but this triggers angiogenesis and release of growth factors, which should increase oxygenation unless other factors are present.

SYSTEMIC FACTORS

Systemic factors that may impact the healing process include:

- **Inadequate nutrition**: A diet with adequate nutrition and protein is necessary for healing, so an inadequate diet may slow the healing process.
- **Obesity**: Patients who are overweight are at increased risk of pressure injuries because of compression of tissues, and have slower rates of healing as well as increased risk of infection.
- **Chronic disease**: Some diseases, such as diabetes mellitus and hypertension may impair healing.
- **Systemic infection**: Whether originating from the wound or elsewhere, a systemic infection impairs healing.
- **Decrease in sex hormones** (usually associated with age): Low levels of androgens and estrogen slow healing of wounds.
- **Stress**: Emotional stress increases glucocorticoids and reduces cytokines at the wound, impairing healing.

Diagnostic Studies

Laboratory Tests Relevant to Wound Healing and Skin Breakdown

Wound healing and the prevention of skin breakdown requires an adequate nutritional status. Labs that assess for malnutrition, anemia, and dehydration are done to assess the risk for skin breakdown and delayed wound healing. Tests that are frequently used as part of wound management include the following.

Total Protein and Albumin

Total protein levels can be influenced by many factors, including stress and infection, but it may be monitored as part of an overall nutritional assessment. Protein is critical for wound healing, and because metabolic rate increases in response to a wound, protein needs increase in wounded patients:

- Normal values: 5-9 g/dL
- Diet requirements for wound healing: 1.25-1.5 g/kg per day

Albumin is a protein that is produced by the liver and is a necessary component for cells and tissues. Levels decrease with renal disease, malnutrition, and severe burns. Albumin levels are the most common screening to determine protein levels. Albumin has a half-life of 18-20 days, so it is more sensitive to long-term protein deficiencies than to short-term.

- Normal values: 3.5-5.5 g/dL
- Mild deficiency: 3-3.5 g/dL
- Moderate deficiency: 2.5-3.0 g/dL
- Severe deficiency: <2.5 g/dL

Levels below 3.2 correlate with increased morbidity and death. Dehydration (poor intake, diarrhea, or vomiting) elevates levels, so adequate hydration is important to ensure meaningful results

Transferrin

Transferrin, which transports about one-third of the body's iron, is a protein produced by the liver. It transports iron from the intestines to the bone marrow where it is used to produce hemoglobin. The half-life of transferrin is about 8-10 days. It is sometimes used as a measure of nutritional status; however, transferrin levels are sensitive to many different things. Levels rapidly decrease with protein malnutrition. Liver disease and anemia can also depress levels, but a decrease in iron, commonly found with inadequate protein, stimulates the liver to produce more transferrin, which increases levels but also decreases production of albumin and prealbumin. Levels may also increase with pregnancy, use of oral contraceptives, and polycythemia. Thus, transferrin levels alone are not always reliable measurements of nutritional status:

- Normal values: 200-400 mg/dL
- Mild deficiency: 150-200 mg/dL
- Moderate deficiency: 100-150 mg/dL
- Severe deficiency: <100 mg/dL

Review Video: Transferrin
Visit mometrix.com/academy and enter code: 267479

Prealbumin

Prealbumin (transthyretin) is most commonly monitored for acute changes in nutritional status because it has a half-life of only 2-3 days. Prealbumin is a protein produced in the liver, so it is often decreased with liver disease. Oral contraceptives and estrogen can also decrease levels. Levels may rise with Hodgkin's disease or the use of steroids or NSAIDS. Prealbumin is necessary for transportation of both thyroxine and vitamin A throughout the body, so if levels fall, both thyroxine and vitamin A utilization are affected.

- Normal values: 16-40 mg/dL
- Mild deficiency: 10-15 mg/dL
- Moderate deficiency: 5-9 mg/dL
- Severe deficiency: <5 mg/dL

Prealbumin is a good measurement because it quickly decreases when nutrition is inadequate and rises quickly in response to increased protein intake. Protein intake must be adequate to maintain levels of prealbumin. Death rates increase with any decrease in prealbumin levels.

Indicators of Hydration

Serum Sodium and Osmolality

Hydration is essential for proper healing and for meaningful results of laboratory measures of nutrition. A number of different tests can be used to monitor hydration.

Serum sodium measures the sodium level in the blood. Some drugs, such as steroids, laxatives, contraceptives, NSAIDS, and IV fluids containing sodium can elevate levels. Other drugs, such as diuretics and vasopressin can reduce levels.

- Normal values: 135-150 mEq/L
- Dehydration: >150 mEq/L

Serum osmolality measures the concentration of ions, such as sodium, chloride, potassium, glucose, and urea, in the blood. Levels increase with dehydration, which stimulates the antidiuretic hormone (AD), resulting in increased water reabsorption and more concentrated urine in an effort to compensate. Changes in osmolality can affect normal cell functioning, eventually destroying the cells if levels remain high.

- Normal levels: 285-295 mOsm/kg H_2O.
- Dehydration: >295 mOsm/kg H_2O.

Blood Urea Nitrogen (BUN), BUN-Creatinine Ratio, and Specific Gravity/Urine

Blood urea nitrogen (BUN), a protein by-product, is excreted by the kidneys. An elevation of both BUN and creatinine indicates kidney disease, but elevated BUN alone may indicate dehydration:

- Normal values: 7-23 mg/dL
- Dehydration: >23 mg/dL

BUN-creatinine ratio monitors renal failure, where there is enhanced reabsorption in the proximal tubules, causing the urea level to rise. Dehydration or conditions that limit fluid into the kidneys increases urea. Increased urea is also an indication of an upper GI bleed where the proteins in the blood are broken down and reabsorbed in the lower intestinal tract.

- Normal value: 10:1
- Dehydration: >25:1

Specific gravity/urine measures the ability of the kidneys to concentrate or dilute the urine according to changes in serum. The most common cause of an increased specific gravity is dehydration. It may also increase with an increased secretion of anti-diuretic hormone (ADH).

- Normal value: 1.003-1.028
- Dehydration: >1.028

GLUCOSE AND HEMOGLOBIN AIC

Glucose is manufactured by the liver from ingested carbohydrates and is stored as glycogen for use by the cells. If intake is inadequate, glucose can be produced from muscle and fat tissue, leading to increased wasting. High levels of glucose are indicative of diabetes mellitus, which predisposes people to skin injuries, slow healing, and infection. Fasting blood glucose levels are used to diagnose and monitor:

- Normal values: 70-99 mg/dL
- Impaired: 100-125 mg/dL
- Diabetes: >125 mg/dL

There are a number of different conditions that can increase glucose levels: stress, renal failure, Cushing syndrome, hyperthyroidism, and pancreas disorders. Medications, such as steroids, estrogens, lithium, phenytoin, diuretics, and tricyclic antidepressants, may increase glucose levels. Other conditions, such as adrenal insufficiency, liver disease, hypothyroidism, and starvation can decrease glucose levels.

Hemoglobin AIC comprises hemoglobin A with a glucose molecule because hemoglobin holds onto excess blood glucose, so it shows the average blood glucose levels over a 2-3 month period and is used primarily to monitor long-term diabetic therapy.

- Normal value: ≤6%
- Elevation: >7%

TOTAL LYMPHOCYTE COUNT

The immune system responds quickly to changes in protein intake because proteins are critical to antibody and lymphocyte production. T lymphocytes develop in the thymus gland and are a part of the cell-mediated immune response. B-lymphocytes develop in the bone marrow and are part of the humoral (antibody-mediated) immune response.

Total lymphocyte count (TLC) can reflect changes in nutritional status because a decrease in protein causes decreased immunity. Lymphocytes are expressed on a differential as a percentage of the white blood count. The TLC is calculated by multiplying the percentage by the total white blood count and then dividing by 100.

- Normal values: 2000 cells/mm^3
- Mild deficiency: 1500-1800 cells/mm^3
- Moderate deficiency: 900-1500 cells/mm^3
- Severe deficiency: <900 cells/mm^3

While low levels may be indicative of malnutrition, levels are also depressed with stress, autoimmune diseases, chemotherapy, infection, and HIV.

COMPLETE BLOOD COUNT WITH RBCS, PLATELETS, HGB AND HCT

The complete blood count with differential and platelet (thrombocyte) count provides information about the blood and other body systems. Red blood cell (erythrocyte) counts and concentrations may vary with anemia, hemorrhage, or various disorders. A decrease in red blood cells may affect healing because of less oxygen to tissues, but changes do not indicate infection.

- **Hemoglobin**, a protein found in erythrocytes, uses iron to bind and transport oxygen. Deficiencies of amino acids, vitamins, or minerals can cause a decrease in hemoglobin, impacting healing and increasing the danger of pressure injuries by reducing oxygen to tissue. Dehydration and severe burns can cause an increase.
    - Normal values: Males, 13-18 g/dL. Females, 12-16 g/dL.

- **Hematocrit** measures the percentage of packed red blood cells in 100 ml of blood. A decrease can indicate blood loss and anemia. An increase may indicate dehydration, and measurements may help to monitor the effects of rehydration.
    - Normal values: Males, 42-52%. Females, 37-48%.
- **Platelet** normal values of 150,000-400,000 may increase to over a million during acute infection.

Complete Blood Count with WBCs and Differential

White blood cell (leukocyte) count is used as an indicator of bacterial and viral infection. WBC is reported as the total number of all white blood cells.

- Normal WBC for adults: 4,800-10,000
- Acute infection: >10,000 (a level of 30,000 or more indicates the infection is severe).
- Viral infection: 4,000 and below

The differential provides the percentage of each different type of leukocyte. An increase in the total white blood cell count is usually related to an increase in one type. Often an increase in immature neutrophils (known as bands) referred to as a "shift to the left," is an indication of an infectious process:

- Normal immature neutrophils (bands): 1-3%. Increase with infection
- Normal segmented neutrophils (segs) for adults: 50-62%. Increase with acute, localized, or systemic bacterial infections.
- Normal eosinophils: 0-3%. Decrease with stress and acute infection.
- Normal basophils: 0-1%. Decrease during acute stage of infection.
- Normal lymphocytes; 25-40%. Increase in some viral and bacterial infections.
- Normal monocytes: 3-7%. Increase during recovery stage of acute infection.

C-Reactive Protein and Erythrocyte Sedimentation Rate

C-reactive protein is an acute-phase reactant produced by the liver in response to an inflammatory response that causes neutrophils, granulocytes, and macrophages to secrete cytokines. Thus, levels of C-reactive protein rise when there is inflammation or infection. It has also been found to be a helpful measurement of response to treatment for pyoderma gangrenosum ulcers:

- Normal values: 2.6-7.6 μg/dL

Erythrocyte sedimentation rate (sed rate) measures the distance erythrocytes fall in a vertical tube of anticoagulated blood in one hour. Because fibrinogen, which increases in response to infection, also increases the rate of the fall, the sed rate can be used as a non-specific test for inflammation when infection is suspected. The sed rate is sensitive to osteomyelitis and may be used to monitor treatment response. Values vary according to gender and age:

- <50: Males 0-15 mm/hr. Females 0-20 mm/hr.
- >50: Males 0-20 mm/hr. Females 0-30 mm/hr.

Wound Culture and Sensitivities

Wound culture and sensitivities are done when there are signs of infection in a wound or no progress in healing over a two-week period. The wound culture identifies the pathogenic agent and the sensitivities show which antimicrobials are the most affective for treatment. The culture should be done prior to the administration of antibiotics, which may interfere with the results. Sterile technique should be used. A culture area may be done, taking the sample from clean tissue rather than exudate, which may give a false report, showing organisms in the area but not in the tissue itself. There are **three methods of culturing**:

- **Swabbing** the area is the most common method used but the sample is easily contaminated by surface flora.
- **Needle aspiration** of fluid adjacent to the wound may result in underestimation of organisms.
- Culturing by **tissue biopsy** is often most effective method, but not all labs can process these samples and the process disrupts the wound and increases pain.

Diagnostic Imaging

Imaging can also be useful when diagnosing and evaluating wounds and vasculature:

- **Magnetic Resonance Angiography (MRA)**: This type of angiography is minimally invasive and may use contrast. Radio waves and a magnetic field produce computer-generated images that are more detailed than with standard angiography.
- **Computed Tomography Angiography (CTA)**: This is a minimally-invasive procedure that may use contrast to enhance vessels. It requires a sophisticated computer program to produce multiple images for computer-generated cross-sectional pictures, but it is becoming more widely available.
- **Computer enhanced angiography**: This is an invasive procedure that requires the insertion of catheters into the femoral artery. Vessel wall injury can occur and clots can be liberated from the vessel walls by accident. The contrast used can damage the kidneys. Angioplasty may be performed during angiography, combining diagnosis with treatment in one procedure. Smaller vessels may not be seen so this test is not conclusive when deciding whether amputation of the limb should take place.

Measuring Venous Refill

Measuring venous refill is critical to diagnosing the cause and wounds and extent/severity of vascular disease:

- **Photo plethysmography (PPG)** measures venous refill time using light absorption via an infrared light emitting diode that emits light through the skin. PPG measures light absorbed and reflected from the hemoglobin of the blood during the filing of tiny blood vessels to determine changes in blood volume.
- **Light Reflective Rheography (LRR)**, based on PPG, uses infrared light and three light diodes, which reduces reflection of external light and the skin surface to produce a more accurate measure of venous refill than the PPG.
- **String Gauge Plethysmography (SGP)** uses PPG to study venous flow, but also uses a string gauge wrapped around the leg to detect tension changes in the calf during exertion, revealing venous refill and emptying.

Determining Adequate Blood Flow

Doppler

Doppler is equipment that provides an ultrasonic evaluation of arterial circulation of the extremities. Doppler evaluation is used when the circulation of the extremity appears impaired (edema, pallor, cyanosis), when pulses cannot be palpated manually, and to determine site for arterial puncture. The procedure is described below:

1. Place conductive gel on the end of the probe or on the skin over the site to be assessed, hold the device at a 45-degree angle to the skin, and move it about the skin until the pulse is heard.
2. Count the pulse rate, describe the intensity, remove the device, wipe away the conductive gel, and then use a marking pen to mark the site.
3. When assessing the sound, the echo heard is at a higher frequency when blood flow is in the direction of the transducer and lower frequency when it is in the opposite direction (representing the Doppler effect/frequency shift).

There are two methods of using doppler to assess blood flow:

- **Continuous wave doppler** is a non-invasive test that uses a pencil-like probe containing a piezoelectric crystal that emits a sound wave that is reflected by the blood vessel back to the probe, producing an audible sound that is analyzed to determine whether blood flow is adequate. The Doppler is also used along with a blood pressure cuff to compare brachial and ankle pressures to diagnose claudication.
- **Laser doppler skin perfusion pressures**: A blood pressure cuff containing a laser probe in the bladder of the cuff is used to measure skin perfusion to detect early limb ischemia. It detects both tissue perfusion and vascular status and is 80% accurate.

Duplex Ultrasound Screening for Lower Extremity Arterial Disease

The purpose of duplex ultrasound screening is to evaluate for the presence of atherosclerotic disease, which causes lower extremity arterial disease. This has traditionally been completed by measuring the ankle-brachial index. Duplex ultrasound of the lower extremity, usually the superficial femoral artery, can be accomplished just as easily and is a more sensitive and specific test to identify for the presence of lower extremity arterial disease. Screening can also help to diagnose early disease, before patients are strongly symptomatic. This could enable them to change any modifiable risk factors, such as smoking or obesity, to decrease their odds of developing strong symptoms or complications of lower extremity arterial disease. This can also be an indicator that there may be coronary artery disease present if the atherosclerotic disease is present in the lower extremity arteries.

Transcutaneous Oxygen Pressure (TcPO$_2$)

Transcutaneous oxygen pressure (TcPO$_2$) uses non-invasive electrodes placed directly on the skin to measure the oxygen being released from the capillaries. These electrodes are heated slightly to ensure blood flow is promoted to the extremity and to minimize misreads secondary to cold-induced vasoconstriction. TcPO$_2$ measurement can be done as an absolute value in mmHg, or as a ratio that compares the value at the extremity to the value at the chest (with 0.9 being accepted as normal). The normal absolute value for perfusion of the lower extremities is around 60 mmHg and a level of >40 mmHg has been proven sufficient for wound healing. When the perfusion level drops below 30 mmHg, healing is compromised. While pulse oximetry is widely used to measure more systemic oxygenation status, TcPO$_2$ is indicated when the goal is to determine the level of ischemia localized to the extremities or to define the severity of vascular compromise or disease. It is often used in measuring perfusion to an amputation site and in managing foot ulcers.

Ultrasound for Monitoring Wound Care and Healing

Ultrasound technology is now used for monitoring wound care and healing as well as promoting healing. Clinical studies are now underway to determine the effectiveness of low-frequency, low-intensity ultrasound treatments for chronic wounds. Some studies indicate that ultrasound stimulation increases the rate of healing. Currently, ultrasound is used primarily for measuring and tracking. For example, Wound Mapping Ultrasound offers three-dimensional measurement, alert notifications, digital imaging, and diagnostic capabilities as well as visualization of blood flow. A special transparent dressing is applied over the wound to protect it from the transducer, so patients may feel pressure or some discomfort. Upon completion of the ultrasound, a report is generated that indicates the size, shape, depth, whether there is undermining or absence presence, and the type of invasion of local tissue that is present (such as to muscle, tendon, bone, and/or joint capsule).

Performing Initial Assessment

Assessing Etiologic Factors

Wounds should be evaluated for **etiology** (the origin of the wound) during the initial assessment to ensure proper treatment. Wounds can arise from a number of different etiologies:

- **Pressure**: Wounds that occur over bony prominences, such as the heels and coccyx, may be related to pressure, shear, or friction. The skin should be carefully examined for discolorations or changes in texture that might indicate compromise.
- **Arterial**: Arterial insufficiency is associated with a decrease in pedal pulses, and cool atrophic (shiny, dry) skin. It may result in small punctate-type ulcers, frequently on the dorsum of foot.
- **Venous stasis**: A decrease in venous circulation often results in hemoglobin leaking into the tissues of the lower leg, causing a brown discoloration. Tissue is often edematous, and ulcers are most common near the medial malleolus.
- **Diabetic neuropathy/ischemia**: Neuropathy can result in a lack of sensation to pain so that injuries to the feet may go unnoticed. Diabetes may also cause damage to small vessels, resulting in ischemia that can lead to ulcerations.
- **Trauma**: Injuries resulting from accidents or other types of trauma may vary considerably with some resulting in extensive damage to bones, tissues, organs, and circulation. Additionally, the wounds may be contaminated. Each wound must be assessed individually for multiple factors.
- **Burns**: Burn wounds may be chemical, thermal, or electric and should be assessed according to the area, the percentage of the body burned, and the depth of the burn.
- **Infection**: An infected surgical or wound site can result in pain, edema, cellulitis, drainage, erosion of the sutures and ulceration of the tissue. Surgical sites must be assessed carefully and laboratory findings reviewed.

Assessing Oxygenation

Assessment of oxygenation includes:

- **Color**: Impaired oxygenation may cause a change in the color of the skin, including pallor and cyanosis, especially in the extremities and about the mouth and nose. Individuals with darker skin may take on a gray, ashy appearance.
- **Respiratory rate**: As oxygenation falls, air hunger may occur with the patient becoming increasingly dyspneic.
- **Oxygen saturation**: While normal oxygen saturation is greater than 95%, as oxygenation is impaired, the level may fall below 92%. Oxygen saturation loses accuracy if the level falls below 80%, so blood gas analysis should be done in those cases.
- **Blood gas analysis**: PO_2 should be greater than 80 mmHg but may fall below 60 mmHg (indicating hypoxemia).
- **Altered mental status**: As oxygen levels fall, the patient may exhibit confusion.
- **Blood lactate level**: Results higher than 2 mEq/L indicate impaired tissue oxygenation.

Neurological/Neurovascular Assessment

Neurological/neurovascular assessment includes:

- **Cranial nerve assessment**: Assess cranial nerves I through VII.
- **Inspection of muscles**: Determine if they are of normal size, strength, and tone and equal bilaterally. Note any involuntary movements (twitches, tremors).
- **Balance assessment**: Assess gait, Romberg test (feet together, eyes closed for 20 seconds), rapid alternating movements, finger-to-finger or finger-to-nose, and heel-to-shin test.
- **Sensory assessment**: Assess spinothalamic tracts for perception of pain, temperature, and light touch. Assess posterior column tract with vibration, position, fine touch, stereognosis, graphesthesia, two-point discrimination, extinction, and point location testing.
- **Reflexes**: Assess deep tendon reflexes (biceps reflex, triceps reflex, brachioradialis reflex, quadriceps reflex, Achilles reflex, and clonus) and superficial cutaneous reflexes (abdominal reflexes, cremasteric reflex, and plantar reflex).
- **Developmental status**: An age-appropriate assessment should determine if the patient's development is within normal parameters. Older adults may exhibit slower response times than younger adults and may exhibit tremors and unsteady gait related to age changes.

Elements of Wound Assessment

Location and Size

Wound location should be described in terms of anatomic position using landmarks (such as sternal notch, umbilicus, lateral malleolus), correct medical terminology, and directional terms:

- Anterior (in front)
- Posterior (behind)
- Superior (above)
- Inferior (below)

Wound size should be carefully described through actual measurement rather than association (the size of a dime). Measurements should be done with a disposable ruler in millimeters or centimeters. The current standard for measurement:

$$\text{length} \times \text{width} \times \text{depth} = \text{dimension}$$

However, a clear description requires more detail. The measurement should be done at the greatest width and greatest length. More than two measurements may be needed if the wound is very irregularly shaped. The depth of the wound should be measured by inserting a sterile applicator and grasping or marking the applicator at skin level and then measuring the length below. Ideally, the wound should be photographed as well, following protocols for photography.

Wound Bed Tissue

Wound bed tissue should be described as completely as possible, including color and general appearance:

- **Granulation tissue** is slightly granular in appearance and deep pink to bright red and moist, bleeding easily if disturbed.
- **Clean non-granular tissue** is smooth and deep pink or red and is not healing.
- **Hypergranulation** is excessive, soft, flaccid granulating tissue that is raised above the level of the periwound tissue, preventing proper epithelization, and may reflect excess moisture in the wound.
- **Epithelization** should appear at wound edges first and then eventually cover the wound. It is dry and light pink or violet in color.
- **Slough** is necrotic tissue that is viscous, soft, and yellow-gray in appearance and adheres to the wound.
- **Eschar** is hard dark brown or black leathery necrotic tissue that accumulates with death of the tissue.

Wound Margins

Wound margins and the tissue surrounding the wound should be described carefully and with correct terminology:

- **Color** should be described using color descriptions and such terms as blanched, erythematous (red), or ecchymosed (purple, green, yellow).
- **Skin texture** may be normal, indurated (hardened), or edematous (swollen). Note if there is cellulitis or maceration evident.
- **Wound edges** may be diffuse (without clear margins), well defined, or rolled. A healing ridge may be evident if granulation has begun. Note if the wound is closed (as with a surgical incision) or open (as with dehiscence or ulcerations). Note if wound edges are attached or unattached (indicating undermining or tunneling).
- **Tunneling or undermining** should be assessed by probing the wound margins with a moist sterile cotton applicator, using clock face locators (toward the head is 12 o'clock, for example). Tunneling may be described as extending from 3 o'clock to 4 o'clock. A large area is usually described as undermining. The size should be measured or estimated as closely as possible.

Distribution, Drainage, and Odor

Distribution of lesions should be clearly delineated if there is more than one lesion over an area. The arrangement of the lesions can be helpful for diagnosis and treatments.

- Linear (in a line)
- Satellites (small lesions around a larger one)
- Diffuse (scattered freely over an area)

Drainage may vary considerably from nothing at all to copious outpourings of discharge.

- Serous drainage is usually clear to slightly yellow.
- Serosanguineous drainage is a combination of serous drainage and blood.
- Sanguineous drainage is bloody.
- Purulent discharge may be thick and milky, yellow, brownish, or green, depending upon the infective agent.

Odor requires more subjective assessment, but the odor and type of discharge together can provide useful information. Some infective agents, such as *Pseudomonas*, produce distinctive odors, which may be described in various ways: musty, foul, sweet.

Wound Exudate

Wound exudate is fluid found in the wound, consisting of blood serum, debris from cells, bacteria, and white blood cells (leukocytes). **Wound exudate** can occur in small to large amounts and, depending on the presence of an organism, may be colored clear or pale yellow (serous), pink or blood tinged (serosanguineous), red (sanguineous), or white/yellow (purulent pus). Consistency can range from thin to milky to thick, and odor may occur. When fluid covers less than one-third of the dressing, it is termed small in amount. Fluid covering one-third to two-thirds of the dressing is considered moderate, and fluid covering over two-thirds of the surface of the dressing is considered large. The presence of exudate can occur when the wound is left untreated or when venous insufficiency, congestive heart failure, malnutrition, kidney or liver disease, or infection is present. One must remember that some odors may be caused by the reaction of the wound fluid on the dressing. Odor can also be caused when the dressing is not changed often enough.

Wound Measurement

Wound measurement determines the progress of healing and must be done accurately and consistently each time. When the wound is a surgical one, it is sufficient to measure length and width, but depth is important for pressure injuries:

- One should use millimeters or centimeters, not inches, in measurement.
- Linear measurement utilizes a plastic or paper ruler marked in centimeters, measuring the greatest length and the greatest width or making the measurements perpendicular to each other. This is the most common method, but it doesn't take into account the shape of the wound and can overestimate the surface area involved when the measurement is multiplied length by width.
- The outline of the wound may also be traced onto an acetate sheet marked in centimeters and the surface area determined by counting the squares.
- Depth is then determined by inserting a sterile moist cotton applicator into the deepest part of the wound.
- Undermining and tunneling tracts are measured in the same manner.

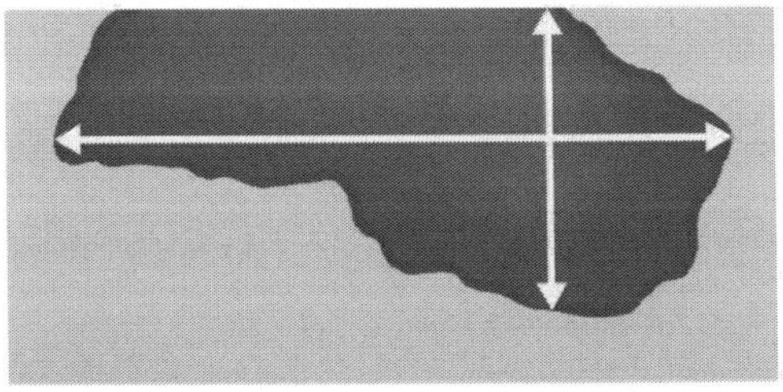

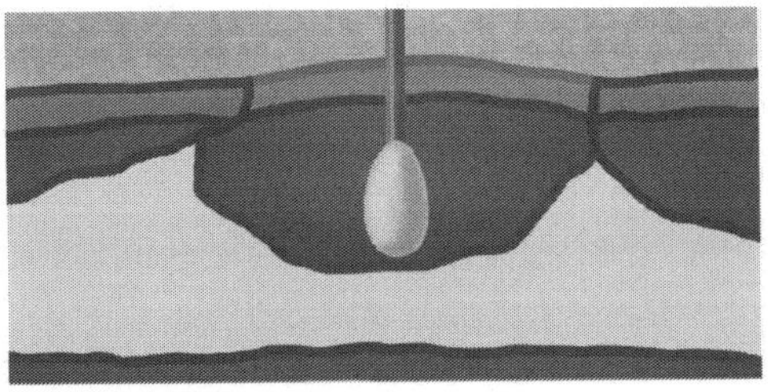

Digital Methods of Wound Measurement

A number of different tools are available for measuring and monitoring wounds using digital equipment. These tools are often more accurate than manual measurements and maintain a historical record that can be easily accessed to track changes. Most tools are software applications that can be loaded onto a smartphone (camera-enabled) or iPad, requiring only that the healthcare provider position the device and take photos. Some programs, such as WoundDesk (Digital MedLab) are primarily management software to improve documentation, but others, such as Scout (WoundVision) provide visual and infrared imaging and both physical and physiological (blood flow, metabolic activity) monitoring. Another program, WoundZoom, contains a 3D sensor and can provide an image of the wound that includes the length, depth, and breadth. Swift Skin and Wound, a widely-used program, offers a wound management system (Swift App for measurement, Swift HealX to calibrate size, color, lighting, and Swift dashboard to display data) that includes wound measurement, imaging, and tracking.

Assessment of Periwound Environment

The periwound environment includes the area around the wound and is an important part of wound assessment:

- Note signs of inflammation such as warmth, erythema, and edema.
- Palpate the skin for firmness and fluctuation that may indicate a subcutaneous abscess.
- Look for signs of breakdown from tape.
- Observe for signs of pale, moist, soft skin that may be maceration caused by exudate from the wound.
- Check the skin for flakiness or evidence of dryness, as the surrounding skin may be too dry if the dressing wicks the moisture out of the skin.
- Examine the skin for signs of circulatory impairment, such as abnormal hair distribution, rubor, or pallor.
- Note evidence of undermining or tunneling that extends under the tissue.

DOCUMENTATION OF THE WOUND ASSESSMENT

The care provider can use the acronym **ASSESSMENT** to help document the thorough assessment of a wound:

- Anatomically locate the wound on the body and include the age of the wound
- Size of the wound in centimeters: length, width, and depth, including shape and stage of the wound
- Sinus tracts, tunneling, fistulas, and undermining at the edges
- Exudate color, amount, and consistency
- Sepsis present in the wound or systemically
- Surrounding skin color, edema, status
- Margins of the wound, attachment to the wound bed, rolling, presence of maceration
- Erythema, presence of epithelialization or eschar
- Necrotic tissue presence, odor of wound, visible blood vessels
- Tissue of wound bed, amount of granulation present, wound tenderness, tension, and temperature

ASSESSMENT CHARACTERISTICS OF ARTERIAL, NEUROPATHIC, AND VENOUS ULCERS

The assessment process is important in delineating between the arterial, neuropathic, or venous origin of the ulcer. Characteristics of each must be known and closely examined:

Location

- **Arterial**: Ends of toes, pressure points, traumatic nonhealing wounds
- **Neuropathic**: Plantar surface, metatarsal heads, toes, and sides of feet
- **Venous**: Between knees and ankles, medial malleolus

Wound Bed

- **Arterial**: Pale, necrotic
- **Neuropathic**: Red (or ischemic)
- **Venous**: Dark red, fibrinous slough

Exudate

- **Arterial**: Slight amount, infection common
- **Neuropathic**: Moderate to large amounts, infection common
- **Venous**: Moderate to large amounts

Wound Perimeter

- **Arterial**: Circular, well-defined
- **Neuropathic**: Circular, well-defined, often with callous formation
- **Venous**: Irregular, poorly-defined

Pain

- **Arterial**: Very painful
- **Neuropathic**: Pain often absent because of reduced sensation
- **Venous**: Pain varies

Skin

- **Arterial**: Pale, friable, shiny, and hairless, with dependent rubor and elevational pallor
- **Neuropathic**: Ischemic signs (as in arterial) may be evident with co-morbidity
- **Venous**: Brownish discoloration of ankles and shin, edema common

Pulses

- **Arterial**: Weak or absent
- **Neuropathic**: Present and palpable, diminished in neuroischemic ulcers
- **Venous**: Present and palpable

Assessing for Wound Complications

Chronic Inflammation

Chronic inflammation of a wound can last for months, delaying wound healing. The immune system may fail to adequately phagocytose debris and dead tissue in the wound and fight infection, and wound care may be inadequate, such as failure to debride the wound or clear infection. Chronic inflammation is caused by debris, necrotic tissue, repeated injury to the wound, and continued effects of histamine release from mast cells. The blood vessels stay dilated, causing warmth, redness, and swelling. The wound-encircling erythema is a ring of redness in light skin or a ring of darkness in dark skin. Pain may be absent or intense if there is infection or arterial vascular disease present. Necrotic tissue may extend over all or part of the wound bed and may be light or dark in color and hard, soft, or stringy. Exudate may be thick, yellow, brown, or green with an odor. The exudate should be cleansed from the wound so that the odor of the wound bed itself can be determined.

Undermining

Undermining occurs at the edges of a wound and may result from shear injuries. The tissues pull away from the base of the wound and a cavity occurs under the intact skin of the wound periphery. The opening of the wound is thus smaller than the area of tissue damage beneath the surface of the skin surrounding the wound. The degree of undermining should be documented by using the face of the clock to describe the location of the undermining in relation to the opening and by recording the depth of the undermining into surrounding tissues by gently probing with a moist sterile cotton applicator. There are two basic **types of undermining**:

- **Initial**: This is related to discharge of liquefied necrotic tissue, leaving undermining that circles the wound. The wound usually lacks signs of epithelialization.
- **Late**: This is related to external pressure (after discharge undermining), and leaves more localized undermining, often in the direction of a bony prominence. The wound shows signs of epithelialization in non-undermined areas.

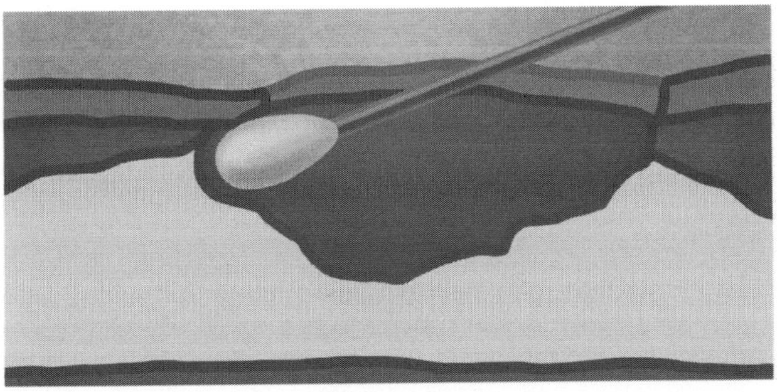

Wound Tunneling

Wound tunneling is a form of undermining that creates a tract that leads away from the wound through subcutaneous tissues between muscles. Tunneling occurs when the fascia that holds muscles together in bundles is cut. Tunneling must be measured with a sterile moist cotton applicator and documented as to depth and width, using the clock face to describe location (3 to 4 o'clock) and then packed loosely to stimulate the healing process. If tunneling ends in a dead space, infection of the wound can progress through the tunnel to cause development of abscess. Tunneling may be caused by infection, pressure that causes tissue necrosis (over bony prominences), or foreign bodies, such as a suture or dressing material left in the wound. It is important for tunnels to heal prior to wound closure to prevent abscess formation, necessitating surgical drainage later. Tunnels are common in surgical wounds in which dehiscence occurs, and the tunnels can join together to form sinus tracts.

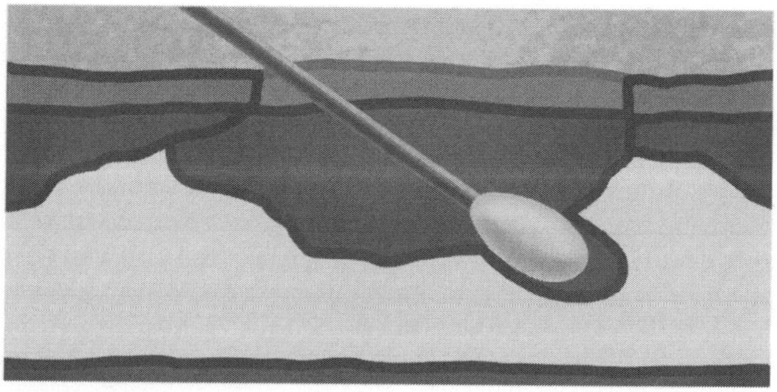

Assessment of Lower Extremities

Assessment of lower extremities includes a number of different elements:

- **Appearance** includes comparing limbs for obvious differences or changes in skin or nails as well as evaluating for edema and color changes in skin, such as pallor or rubor.
- **Perfusion** should be assessed by checking venous filling time, capillary refill, skin temperature (noting changes in one limb or between limbs), bruits (indicating arterial narrowing), pulses (comparing both sides in a proximal to distal progression), ankle-brachial index, and toe-brachial index.
- **Sensory function** includes the ability to feel pain, temperature, and touch.
- **Range of motion** of the ankle must be assessed to determine if the joint flexes past 90° because this is necessary for unimpaired walking and aids venous return in the calf.
- **Pain** is an important diagnostic feature of peripheral arterial disease, so the location, intensity, duration, and characteristics of pain are important.

Pulse

Evaluation of the pulses of the lower extremities is an important part of assessment for peripheral arterial disease. Pulses should be first evaluated with the patient in supine position and then again with the legs dependent, checking bilaterally and proximally to distally to determine if intensity of pulse decreases distally. The pulse should be evaluated as to rate, rhythm, and intensity, which is usually graded on a 0-4 scale:

0 = pulse absent
1 = weak, difficult to palpate
2 = normal as expected
3 = full
4 = strong and bounding

Pulses may be palpable or absent with peripheral arterial disease. Absence of pulse on both palpation and Doppler probe does indicate peripheral arterial disease.

Procedure and Sites for Pulse Checks

Pulses can be assessed in the following order at the following sites:

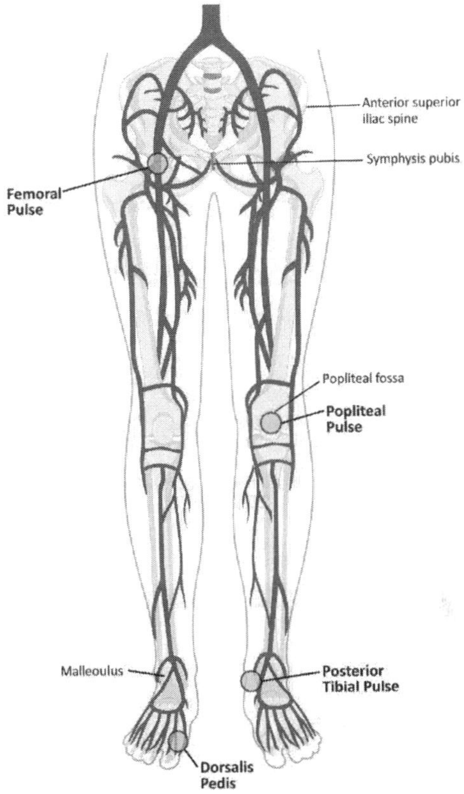

- Beginning with the **dorsalis pedis** (on the top of the foot), palpate above the toes between the great and second toe and move upward until the pulse is palpable.
- Next, assess the **posterior tibial pulse**, which is located on the medial side of the ankle behind and slightly below the malleolus.
- Moving up the leg, the **popliteal pulse** should be assessed:
  - Ask the patient to place the leg straight and relax the leg.
  - Grasp the knee with both hands with thumbs on the sides of the knees, feeling for the pulse in the popliteal fossa.
- The **femoral pulse** is often difficult to assess in adults because the artery lies deep:
  - Apply deep pressure midway between the symphysis pubis and the anterior superior iliac spine.

Bruit

Bruits (a sound indicating turbulent blood flow through a vessel) may be noted by auscultating over major arteries, such as femoral, popliteal, peroneal, and dorsalis pedis. Bruits often indicate peripheral arterial disease.

Perfusion

Assessment of perfusion can indicate venous or arterial abnormalities:

- **Venous refill time**: Begin with the patient lying supine for a few moments and then have the patient sit with the feet dependent. Observe the veins on the dorsum of the foot and count the seconds before normal filling. Venous occlusion or arterial supply inadequacy is indicated with times >20 seconds.
- **Capillary refill**: Grasp the toenail bed between the thumb and index finger and apply pressure for several seconds to cause blanching. Release the nail and count the seconds until the nail regains normal color. Arterial occlusion/insufficiency is indicated with times >2-3 seconds. Checks both feet and more than one nail bed.
- **Skin temperature**: Using the palm of the hand and fingers, gently palpate the skin, moving distally to proximally and comparing both legs. Arterial disease is indicated by decreased temperature (coolness) or a marked change from proximal to distal. Venous disease is indicated by increased temperature about the ankle.

ABI

The ankle-brachial index (ABI) examination is done to evaluate peripheral arterial disease of the lower extremities.

1. Apply a blood pressure cuff to one arm, palpate brachial pulse, and place conductivity gel over the artery.
2. Place the tip of a Doppler device at a 45-degree angle into the gel at the brachial artery and listen for the pulse sound.
3. Inflate the cuff until the pulse sound ceases and then inflate 20 mmHg above that point.
4. Release air and listen for the return of the pulse sound. This reading is the brachial systolic pressure.
5. Repeat the procedure on the other arm, and use the higher reading for calculations.
6. Repeat the same procedure on each ankle with the cuff applied above the malleoli and the gel over the posterior tibial pulse to obtain the ankle systolic pressure.
7. Divide the ankle systolic pressure by the brachial systolic pressure to obtain the ABI.

Sometimes, readings are taken both before and after 5 minutes of walking on a treadmill.

INTERPRETING RESULTS

Once the ankle-brachial index (ABI) examination is completed, the ankle systolic pressure must be divided by the brachial systolic pressure. Ideally, the blood pressure at the ankle should be equal to that of the arm or be slightly higher. With peripheral arterial disease, the ankle pressure falls, lowering the ABI. Additionally, some conditions that cause calcification of arteries, such as diabetes, can cause a false elevation. Calculation of the ABI ratio is simple: divide the ankle systolic BP by brachial systolic BP. For example, if the ankle BP is 90 and the brachial BP is 120, the ABI ratio is:

$$90 \div 120 = 0.75$$

The degree of disease relates to the ABI ratio as follows:

- >1.4 Abnormally high, may indicate calcification of vessel wall
- 1.0-1.4: Normal reading, asymptomatic
- 0.9-1.0: Low, but acceptable unless there are other indications of PAD
- 0.8-0.9: Likely some arterial disease is present
- 0.4-0.7 Moderate arterial disease
- <0.4 Severe arterial disease

TOE-BRACHIAL INDEX

The procedure for toe-brachial index (TBI) is as follows:

1. Apply blood pressure cuff to one arm, palpate brachial pulse, and place conductivity gel over the artery.
2. Place the tip of a Doppler device at a 45-degree angle into the gel at the brachial artery and listen for the pulse sound.
3. Inflate the cuff until the pulse sound ceases and then inflate 20 mmHg above that point.
4. Release air and listen for the return of the pulse sound. This reading is the brachial systolic pressure.
5. Repeat the procedure on the other arm and use the higher reading for calculations.
6. Repeat the same procedure on the great or second toe with the cuff applied around the base of the toes and the gel over the pulse to obtain the toe systolic pressure.
7. Divide the toe systolic pressure by the brachial systolic pressure to obtain the TBI (same calculations as for ABI). Normal values are >0.6.

Assessing the Gaiter Area and for Hemosiderin Staining

Two common signs of venous insufficiency that must be assessed in the lower extremities include:

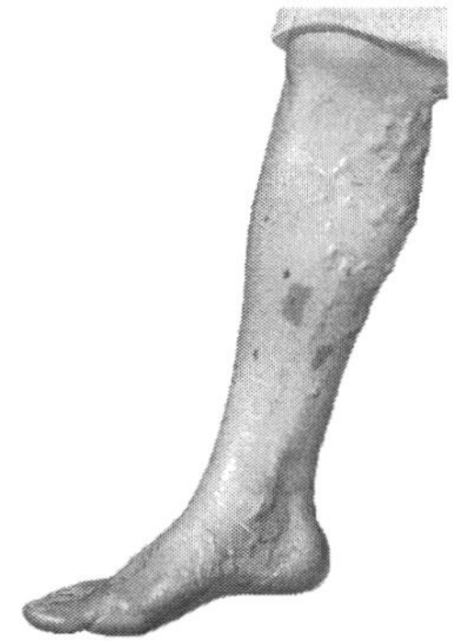

- **Gaiter area:** The region of the leg between the knee and ankle. This is the area in which most venous ulcers occur. Venous ulcers are commonly found around the medial or lateral malleoli within this region and tend to be large, shallow, and not painful. The wound bed is usually filled with irregular granulation tissue. Within this area, it is also common to see varicose veins and stasis dermatitis changes, as shown here.
- **Hemosiderin staining:** When a patient has a venous ulcer, there is frequently bleeding into the surrounding tissues. The blood cells break down in the tissues and their contents are absorbed by macrophages. The hemoglobin within red blood cells is broken down, and the iron within this is combined with proteins and changed into a stored form of iron. This stored form of iron contains a dark pigment called hemosiderin, which will give the patient a hyperpigmented area of skin. Patients frequently confuse this for a bruised area, though it may take years for the body to absorb this stored form of iron.

Assessing for Peripheral Neuropathy

Nylon Monofilament Test

A simple test for peripheral neuropathy, commonly used to determine risk of ulcers in diabetic patients, is the nylon monofilament test, which is available in kits:

1. Describe the procedure to the patient and ask the patient to indicate when the pressure of the monofilament is felt.
2. Grasp a length of #10 monofilament in the instrument provided.
3. Touch the monofilament against the bottom of the foot, and then press the monofilament into the foot until the line buckles.
4. Test the great, 3rd, and 5th toes.
5. Test the left, medial, and right areas of the ball of the foot.
6. Test the right and left of the arch.
7. Test the middle of the heel.

The test is evaluated according to how many of the 10 test sites the patient is able to detect. If the patient fails to detect the monofilament at fewer than 4 sites, this is indicative of decreased sensation and increased risk.

Sensory Vibration Testing

Sensory vibration testing is done with a tuning fork when a patient has a normal monofilament exam of the foot but still may be at risk for foot problems because of reduced sensation, especially patients with diabetes. To carry out the exam, the patient is placed in supine position with the feet exposed. Tap the tuning fork against the ball of the hand and then place the tip of the tuning fork against the bone near the end of the big toe, below the nail, or on top of the great toe joint. Ask the patient to indicate when the feeling of vibration stops. Both the examiner and the patient should feel the vibration stop at the same time if the patient has normal sensation. If the patient doesn't feel the vibration or feels it stop before the examiner, calculate the difference in seconds. Test both feet and note any differences.

ASSESSMENT OF LEND LEADING TO NEUROPATHIC/DIABETIC WOUNDS

The assessment for lower extremity neuropathic disease (LEND) and neuropathic/diabetic wounds includes:

- **History***:* A history of general health and record of diabetes control and complications is critical. Risk factors should be identified and risks classified according to severity.
- **Physical examination***:* The examination must identify any co-morbid conditions, such as heart disease, arthritis, and peripheral arterial or venous insufficiency.
- **Lower extremity/foot examination***:* A thorough examination of the lower extremity and foot should include screening for neuropathy and sensory loss, pain, musculoskeletal changes or abnormalities, and vascular status. The skin should be carefully assessed for corns, calluses, pre-ulcerative lesions (such as blisters or cracks). Nails should be checked for fungus infections and thickening, which is common, and discolorations, such as red, black, or brown that may indicate trauma. Footwear should be examined for support and fit.
- **Evaluation and classification of the diabetic foot ulcer (DFU):** Ulcers should be measured and classified according to standard classification systems, observing for signs of infection.

ASSESSING ADEQUACY OF FOOTWEAR FOR THOSE WITH LEND

Examining footwear to determine if the fit is correct and if they are appropriate:

- **Examine shoes and slippers** for bulges on the side that may indicate the shoes are too tight, wear patterns on the shoes or heels that may indicate uneven gait or weight distribution. Check inside the shoes to see if there is worn or torn lining that could irritate the skin. Make sure that there is adequate cushioning. Sandals and open-toed shoes should be avoided because of the potential for foot injury.
- **Foot imprints***:* Using the Harris Mat, the patient steps down barefoot on the mat that creates a visual (inked) image of the foot, showing pressure areas with darker images. It shows areas of the foot at greatest risk.
- **Forefoot test***:* An outline of both bare feet is traced on paper while the patient is standing if possible. Then the shoes are placed over this and another outline drawn. The entire foot outline should be inside the shoe outline.

ASSESSMENT FOR FOOT DEFORMITIES RELATED TO DIABETIC ULCERS

The assessment for foot deformities related to diabetic ulcers is described below:

- Inflammation of connective tissue from the heel to ball of foot:
  - Plantar fasciitis—causes severe heel pain
- Bony heel growths:
  - Heel spurs—abnormal protruding growths of bone on the calcaneus, leading to plantar fasciitis.
- Distal muscle atrophy:
  - Hammer toe (contracture of proximal joint of toe)
  - Mallet toe (contracture of distal joint of toe)
  - Claw toe (contracture of both joints of toe)
- Changes in metatarsal bones:
  - Metatarsal bones lower or longer than adjoining bones uneven weight distribution, resulting in pain and ulceration
  - Bunion (enlargement of first metatarsal bone below first toe)

- Arch changes:
  - High cramped instep (*pes cavus*)
  - Flat foot (*pes planus*)
- Weakening of dorsum/plantar surfaces:
  - Charcot's arthropathy—involves weakened bones fracturing and the foot changing shape and becoming inflamed as the arch collapses, causing the foot to have a convex shape
- Nerve irritation:
  - Neuromas between toes

ASSESSMENT OF EDEMA

Edema is usually assessed by pressing the index finger into the tissue on top of each foot, behind the medial malleolus, and over the shin, starting distally and moving proximally to the highest level of edema, comparing both legs: Edema is rated on a 1- to 4-point scale:

- 1+ Slight pitting to about 2 mm; rebounds immediately.
- 2+ Moderate pitting to about 4 mm; rebounds in less than 15 seconds.
- 3+ Moderate-severe pitting to about 6 mm; rebounds in 15-30 seconds.
- 4+ Severe pitting to 8 mm or more; rebounds in greater than 30 seconds.

Types of edema:

- **Venous edema**: Edema from ankle to knee and may involve some limitation in ankle movement. Dependent pitting edema occurs, but may become non-pitting in chronic disease.
- **Lymphedema**: Usually unilateral non-pitting hard edema from toes to groin or fingers to axilla. In advanced disease, elephantiasis with huge enlargement of extremity may occur.
- **Lipedema**: Symmetrical bilateral soft rubbery tissue from ankle to groin and sometimes hips with pain on palpation and frequent bruising.

LIMB VOLUME MEASUREMENTS

Limb volume measurements are used primarily to assess muscle mass growth, assess peripheral edema, and evaluate lymphedema. Comparison is often done with an opposite limb. Methods utilized for limb volume measurements include:

- **Water displacement**: This method (inserting the limb into a container with a measured volume of water and then measuring the overflow water) enables a more accurate volume measurement of hands and feet but cannot be used with open wounds. It provides volume but no information about shape or condition. Additionally, it is difficult to do with full limbs.
- **Circumferential**: Skin markings are placed distally to proximally every 4 cm for the hand and arm and every 10 cm for the foot and leg. Foot should be in dorsiflexion position and hand flat. Measurements are taken and recorded at each mark, avoiding tension on the measuring tape. Tables are available to help calculate the volume based on the tape measurements.
- **Perometer**: Equipment that uses an infrared laser system to read limb measurements and software to calculate limb volume.

Management of Edema

Chronic venous insufficiency (CVI) results in edema of the lower extremities, causing both discomfort and increased risk of ulcers. Treatment includes:

- **Leg elevation** when sitting to avoid dependency. Therapy may include lying down and elevating the affected limb above the heart for 1-2 hours two times daily and during the night. This is important for all patients with CVI, but especially for those unable to comply with compression therapy.
- **Compression therapy** can be used to suit the patient's specific clinical needs, based on mobility status, exercise needs, optimal pressure, and the available assistance they have to help with changing bandages or stockings. Common compression methods include elastic bandages, non-elastic bandages, multicomponent bandage systems, compression stockings, and intermittent pneumatic compression devices.
- **Surgical intervention** is indicated if more conservative treatment is unsuccessful in managing CVI.
- **Ligation and stripping** removes a vein or section of a vein that is damaged or has damaged valves. An incision below the vein allows an endoscope to be threaded into the vein to grasp and remove (strip) it. The vein is tied (ligated). Sometimes only ligation of a faulty valve is done and the vein is left in place.
- **Deep vein reconstruction** may be considered if other approaches fail.
- **Physical therapy** is important because effective calf muscle pumping requires ankle mobility with dorsiflexion over 90°. Some patients may benefit from gait training and exercises to improve the range of motion and strength of the ankle. Calf muscle exercises may include isotonic exercises. Patients need to alternate sitting and standing with walking on a regular schedule throughout the day.
- **Control of weight** often improves circulation and reduces edema, as obesity may be the primary cause of the circulatory impairment. Patients may need education and referral to a bariatric treatment center.
- **Medications** cannot correct venous insufficiency but some can help to control symptoms:
    - Pentoxifylline (Trental) enhances blood flow in capillaries.
    - Horse chestnut seed extract (HCSE) results in reduced pain and edema. It is widely used in Europe and has been studied in the United States. One problem is that it can cause low blood glucose levels in children and those with diabetes.

Lymphedema

Lymphedema is a dysfunction of the lymphatic system, resulting in a debilitating progressive disease. The healthy lymphatic system returns proteins, lipids, and fluids to the circulatory system from the interstitial spaces, but with lymphedema this accumulates, causing pronounced induration, edema, and fibrosis of tissues. As the fluid builds up, it causes distention, and the skin becomes thick and fibrotic with dimpling similar to that of an orange peel (peau d'orange). Scaly keratinous debris collects, and the skin develops cracks and leakage of lymphatic fluid. Lymphedema may be primary (developmental abnormality) or secondary. It can occur after mastectomy, radiation, infection, cancer, or surgery, such as joint replacements and vascular procedures. Patients are at risk of infection, cellulitis, and lymphangitis, as well as pain and limited mobility. Lymphedema has three **stages**:

- Stage 1 is reversible pitting edema distally with no fibrosis.
- Stage 2 is pitting or non-pitting edema with fibrosis and papillomatosis.
- Stage 3 is elephantiasis with massive enlargement and distortion of limb, fibrosis, and ulcerations.

MEDICAL MANAGEMENT

Medical management of lymphedema is intended to reduce the protein accumulation in the tissues and restore lymphatic circulation, but treatment needs to begin before extensive fibrosis occurs. Diuretics do not help and the treatments must be continued lifelong in order to be successful:

- Skin must be kept clean and dry and inspected for open areas or signs of infection. Mild emollients may improve skin barrier.
- Antimicrobial or antifungal topical agents are used for infections. About 15-25% requires long-term antibiotic prophylaxis.
- Limbs need to be elevated when possible during the day and always at night.
- Complex decongestive therapy with massage helps improve lymphatic drainage.
- Static compression bandaging during the day, providing 40-60 mmHg pressure. The bandaging may be removed at night if the limb is elevated.
- Dynamic compression (intermittent dynamic compression) may be used but can displace fluid or further damage lymphatics if not monitored carefully.
- Weight loss may be advised because obesity further compromises lymphatic circulation.

PATIENT MANAGEMENT

Because management of lymphedema is a lifelong process, compliance on the part of the patient is critical to controlling lymphedema and preventing further deterioration and complications. The patient must take an active role:

- Avoid excessive heat, such as sun exposure, saunas, and hot tubs.
- Use an electric razor instead of a straight razor or chemicals for hair removal to prevent injury to skin.
- Prevent trauma to limb. Wear protective gloves and clothing to prevent trauma to affected limb. Avoid blood tests or blood pressure readings in an affected arm.
- Observe skin carefully for signs of cellulitis or infection and follow prescribed protocols for treatment.
- Maintain good hygiene.
- Wear closed-toe shoes if lower limb is affected.
- Use sunscreen and bug repellent on affected limb.
- Avoid lifting and limit use of affected arm.

NUTRITIONAL FACTORS THAT AFFECT THE SKIN

Nutritional status is very important for maintaining the integrity of the skin:

- People who are on restrictive diets or do not have adequate protein in their diets will lack the amino acids for protein synthesis.
- A diet too low in fats can be deficient in essential fatty acids, which the skin cells need for the lipid barrier.
- Carbohydrates are necessary for the cell to carry out basic metabolic functions.
- Vitamin A helps to repair skin tissue.
- Vitamin B complex, especially biotin, is critical for skin formation and prevents dryness and itching.
- Vitamins C and E have been shown to reduce and counter the negative effects of ultraviolet radiation caused by exposure to the sun. Since Vitamin C is utilized for collagen formation, it is essential that intake is adequate.
- Minerals, such as iron, selenium, zinc, and copper are important also.

Initial Nutritional Assessment

Nutritional assessment should be done within the first 24 hours of care to ensure that nutritional requirements of the patient are met. The history and physical exam should include the following information about the **previous three months**:

- Changes in food intake, including number of meals eaten daily
- Weight loss (or gain)
- Episodes of depression or stress that may relate to dietary intake
- A sample of a usual daily menu

Additional screening should include:

- Daily number of proteins, fruit, grain, and vegetable servings
- Usual fluid intake, including type, amount, and frequency
- Method of feeding, independent or assisted
- Mobility
- Mental status
- Body mass index (BMI), mid-arm circumference, and calf circumference
- Living status (independent or dependent)
- Prescription and non-prescription drugs
- Pressure sores or other wounds or skin problems

Nutritional Assessment Tools

Standardized nutritional assessment tools include the following:

- **The MNA (Mini-Nutritional Assessment)** by Nestle Nutrition is designed for nutritional assessment of those over age 65 and is only valid for that population. It is a screening and assessment tool to determine the risk for malnutrition and comprises 15 questions about dietary habits and 4 measurements, including BMI using height and weight, and mid-arm and calf circumference.
- **The Nutritional Screening Initiative** is another tool for geriatric patients and screens for dietary information as well as social and environmental factors, such as whether the person eats alone, prepares meals, drinks alcohol, and has sufficient income.
- **The Subjective Global Assessment** assesses nutritional status by a thorough history and physical examination. The history assesses weight change, dietary intake, gastrointestinal symptoms, and functional impairment. The results of this assessment tool are evaluated subjectively and scores assigned to determine if malnutrition risks are normal to severe.

Physical Assessment of Nutrition

Indications of Nutritional Deficiency

The physical assessment is an important part of nutritional assessment to determine **malnutrition** or problems with **self-feeding**.

- **Hair** may be dry and brittle or thinning.
- **Skin** may show poor turgor, ecchymosis, tears, pressure areas, ulcerations, abrasions, or other compromises.
- The **mouth** may show dry mucous membranes. Lips may be scaly (riboflavin deficiency), have cheilosis, and be cracking at the corners. Gums may be swollen or bleeding, teeth loose or needing care, or dentures poorly fitting. The tongue may be inflamed, dry, cracked, or have sores.
- **Nails** may become brittle. Spoon-shaped or pale nail bed indicates low iron.
- **Hands** may be crippled or arthritic, making eating difficult.
- **Vision** may be compromised so that people can't see to prepare food or have difficulty feeding themselves.
- **Mental status** may be impaired to the point that people can't understand diet instructions or prepare or eat meals.
- **Motor skills** may decrease, including hand-mouth coordination or the ability to hold utensils.

TST, MAC, and MAMC Measurement

Certain measurements aid in the diagnosis of weight- and nutrition-related disorders:

- **Triceps skinfold thickness (TST)** is measured using special calipers. The midpoint between the axilla and elbow of the non-dominant arm is measured and located, and then the skin is grasped between the thumb and index finger about 1 cm above the midpoint at the edges of the arm. The finger and thumb are moved inward until a firm fold of tissue is observed. The calipers are placed about this fold at the midpoint (right below the fingers) and squeezed for 3 seconds, and then a measurement is taken to the nearest millimeter. Three readings are taken with the average of the three used as the measurement.
- **Mid-arm circumference (MAC)** measurement is obtained by measuring in centimeters at the midpoint between the axilla and elbow.
- **Mid-arm muscle circumference (MAMC)** is calculated by multiplying the triceps skinfold thickness (in millimeters) by pi (3.14), and subtracting the result from the mid-arm circumference with results in centimeters.

Triceps skinfold thickness (TST) evaluates fat stores, which often change slowly, so this is not a sensitive test for malnutrition, but it can be used to determine if fat is increasing while muscle mass is decreasing. Mid-arm circumference (MAC) measures muscles, bones, and skin, and mid-arm muscle circumference (MAMC) measures lean body mass. These vary considerably from person to person so they are more useful for tracking muscle wasting over time than for comparisons between different individuals. The TST, MAC, and MAMC are recorded as a percentage of standard measurements, which are quantified for males and females.

- Males
  - TST: 12.5 mm
  - MAC: 29.9 cm
  - MAMC: 25.3 cm
- Females
  - TST: 16.5 mm
  - MAC: 28.5 cm
  - MAMC: 23.3 cm

In order to reach the percentage, the actual measurement for each test is divided by the standard measurement, and that result is multiplied by 100. Thus, if a male's TST measured 11.8:

$$11.8 \div 12.5 = 0.944 \times 100 = 94.4\%$$

BMI

The body mass index (BMI) formula is a measurement that uses height and weight as an indicator of obesity/malnutrition. This cannot be used alone to diagnose obesity as body types differ considerably. Women often have more body fat than men. Tables are available to make calculations simple, but the BMI can be calculated manually:

BMI formula using pounds and inches:

$$\text{BMI} = \frac{\text{weight in pounds} \times 703}{(\text{height in inches})^2}$$

BMI formula using kilograms and meters:

$$\text{BMI} = \frac{\text{weight in kilograms}}{(\text{height in meters})^2}$$

Resulting scores for adults age 20 and over are interpreted according to this chart:

- Below 18.5: Underweight
- 18.5-24.9: Normal weight
- 25.0-29.9: Overweight
- 30 and above: Obese

BMI for those under age 20 uses age-gender specific charts provided by the CDC, containing a curved line that indicates percentiles. The criteria for obesity based on these charts and BMI for age are as follows:

- $<5^{th}$ percentile: Underweight
- 85th-<95 percentile: At risk for overweight
- $>95^{th}$ percentile: Overweight

Waist Hip Ratio

The Waist Hip Ratio (WHR) is the ratio of fat stored about the abdomen and the fat stored around the hips. This ratio is considered of increasing import because an increase in this ratio is associated with increased risk of heart disease, brain attacks, and diabetes mellitus. The formula:

$$\mathbf{WHR} = \frac{\text{waist circumference in centimeters}}{\text{hip circumference in centimeters}}$$

The waist measurement is taken at the smallest circumference, usually slightly above the umbilicus, and the hip measurement at the widest part of the hips, usually about 7 inches below the waist.

The results of the calculation provide a score with risks according to gender:

- Males: WHR >1 means increased risk
- Females: WHR >0.85 means increased risk

Studies have indicated that people who carry more weight around their waists relative to their hips (apple-shaped) are more at risk for complications related to weight than those that carry more weight in their hips (pear-shaped).

Measuring Head Circumference to Assess Nutrition

Head circumference measurements are taken for children during the first 3 years. While there can be non-nutritional reasons for decreased growth of the head, it can also be a sign of a severe lack of nutrition and may be associated with decreased linear growth as well. The measurement is obtained through the following steps:

1. Use non-stretchable measuring tape.
2. Child should be standing or held in sitting position with head upright.
3. Place tape around head just above the eyebrows in the font and around the occipital area in the back.
4. Take at least 3 readings or more until 2 measurements are within 0.1 cm.
5. Use growth chart to determine if measurement is within normal limits.

The CDC provides growth charts for both head circumference and linear growth that are specific for gender, showing the percentile ranking of measurements. Evaluation depends upon various factors, including results of height and weight measurement, to determine if a child is undernourished. Findings below the 5th percentile are usually cause for concern.

Malnutrition

Risk Factors and Indicators for Malnutrition

There are a number of risk factors for malnutrition:

- **Hypermetabolism** resulting from various diseases such as AIDS, as well as trauma, stress, or infection
- **Weight loss**, especially sudden or loss of 10% of normal weight over a 3-month period
- **Low body weight** of <90% of ideal body weight for age or **low body mass index** (BMI) <18.5
- **Immunosuppressive drugs** that interfere with absorption of nutrients
- **Malabsorption** of nutrients caused by diseases, such as chronic failure of kidneys or liver
- **Changes in appetite** that decrease intake of nutrients
- **Food intolerances**, such as lactose intolerance, resulting from lack of enzymes needed to completely digest food so it can be absorbed into the blood stream from the small intestine
- **Dietary restrictions**, such as the limiting of protein with kidney failure
- **Functional limitations**, such as an inability to feed oneself
- **Lack of teeth or dentures**, limiting intake
- **Alterations of taste or smell** that render food unpalatable

Types of Malnutrition and Symptoms

Protein malnutrition (kwashiorkor or hypoalbuminemia) is characterized by inadequate protein but adequate fats and carbohydrates. It can result from chronic diarrhea, renal disease, infection, hemorrhage, burns, traumatic injuries, or other illnesses. Onset is usually rapid with loss of visceral protein while skeletal muscle mass is retained, so it may be difficult to detect on a physical exam. Symptoms include:

- Hypoalbuminemia and anemia
- Edema
- Delayed healing of wound
- Immuno-incompetence

Protein-calorie malnutrition (marasmus), inadequate protein and calories, is usually more obvious. Visceral protein is usually intact, as is immune function, because weight loss is gradual. However, patients are often very thin or emaciated from loss of skeletal muscle mass. Many are elderly and have chronic illnesses. Symptoms include:

- Decreased basal metabolism
- Lack of subcutaneous fat
- Tissue turgor
- Bradycardia
- Hypothermia

Mixed protein-calorie malnutrition (combination) is common in hospitalized patients and has an acute onset with low visceral protein as well as rapid loss of weight, skeletal muscle mass, and fat.

Starvation and Excessive Intake

In response wounds, the stress response causes a hypermetabolic state, and caloric and protein needs increase markedly at the same time intake decreases, leading to periods of **starvation**:

- A **short period** can result in increased nitrogen in urine and increased output with a rapid loss of muscle and weight.
- A **prolonged period** results in slower weight and muscle loss but can lead to metabolic acidosis with increased ammonia in urine and decreased nitrogen.
- An **extended period** becomes premorbid with obvious cachexia and weight loss. The mid-arm muscle circumference decreases and there is increase in creatinine/height index and urinary urea as well as decrease in serum albumin, transferrin, and lymphocytes.

Excessive intake may cause obesity, which delays wound healing, but it does not necessarily mean nutrition is adequate. Overweight people can still have inadequate protein, vitamins, and minerals. Because protein and caloric requirements for healing are tied to weight, nutritional needs are high, but fat stores help people to tolerate prolonged periods of starvation.

Nociceptive Pain

There are two primary types of pain: nociceptive (acute) pain and neuropathic (chronic) pain although some people may have a combination. **Nociceptive** or acute pain is the normal nerve response to a painful stimulus. Trauma that results in nociceptive pain can cause severe inflammation and damage to nerve endings. Nociceptive pain usually correlates with extent and type of injury: the greater the injury, the greater the pain. It may be procedural pain (related to wound manipulation and dressing changes) or surgical pain (related to cutting of tissue). It may also be continuous or cyclic, depending upon the type of injury. This type of pain is usually localized to the area of injury and resolves over time as healing takes place. This type of pain is often described as aching or throbbing, but generally responds to analgesia. Uncontrolled, this type of pain can result in changes in the nervous system that lead to chronic neuropathic pain.

Neuropathic Pain

Neuropathic or chronic pain occurs when there is a primary lesion in the nervous system or dysfunction related to damaged nerve fibers. Neuropathic pain may be associated with conditions such as diabetes, cancer, or traumatic injury to the nervous system. This type of pain is common in chronic wounds and is more often described as burning, stabbing, electric, or shooting pains. Often the underlying pathology causing the pain is not reversible. Pain may be **visceral** (diffuse or cramping pain of internal organs) caused by injuries to internal organs. It is also often diffuse rather than localized. It may also be **somatic pain** (involving muscles, skin, bones, and joints). Neuropathic pain is often more difficult to assess that nociceptive pain because the damage may alter normal pain responses. Neuropathic pain often responds better to antidepressants and anti-seizure medications than analgesics.

Consequences of Pain

Part of managing pain is understanding patients' perceptions regarding pain and its consequences. Some expect and accept pain, and some lack the cognizant awareness to express that they are in pain. Pain, however, is very debilitating and limits quality of life for many patients:

- **Limited activity**: Patients may be unable to stand, walk, or do their jobs, resulting in their being more sedentary, impairing circulation.
- **Frustration**: Acute or chronic pain can lead to depression and anger, as well as withdrawal from activities or lack of desire to try new activities. Patients may withdraw from friends and family.

Additionally, pain has **physiological consequences**:

- **Wound care**: Adequate care of the wound may be limited by pain during treatment. Patients may not carry out prescribed treatments or may refuse treatments.
- **Perfusion**: Pain can result in peripheral vasoconstriction, decreasing perfusion of tissue and impairing leukocyte activity. This depresses angiogenesis, further impairing healing of the wound and continuing the cycle of pain.

Pain Assessment Methods

Pain is subjective and may be influenced by the individual's pain threshold (the smallest stimulus that produces the sensation of pain) and pain tolerance (the maximum degree of pain that a person can tolerate). The most common current **pain assessment tool** is the 1-10 scale:

- 0 = no pain
- 1-2 = mild pain
- 3-5 = moderate pain
- 6-7 = severe pain
- 8-9 = very severe pain
- 10 = excruciating pain

However, there is more to pain assessment than a number on a scale. Assessment includes information about **onset, duration, and intensity**. Identifying what **triggers** pain and what **relieves** it can be very useful when developing a plan for pain management. Patients may show very different **behavior** when they are in pain. Some may cry and moan with minor pain, and others may exhibit seemingly normal behavior even when truly suffering; thus, judging pain by behavior can lead to the wrong conclusions.

Assessing Activities in Relation to Pain

Assessment of pain must include determining those factors or activities that increase pain:

- **Site of pain**: While pain is often focused on the wound site, it may extend to the surrounding tissues, especially in chronic wounds, making application and removal of dressings especially painful.
- **Movement**: Pressure and touch caused by changes of position can increase pain, limiting mobility.
- **Time**: Pain often increases at night, making sleep difficult.
- **Dressings**: Dressings that are too tight or the wrong choice for a wound may cause intense site pain. Allowing the wound to become dry can also increase pain.
- **Personal/cultural**: Some people have difficulty expressing the degree of pain. Others react to the expectation of the medical personnel or family. Some believe that they should remain stoic or are afraid of becoming "addicted," so they resist taking pain medications until pain is severe.

Patients with Impaired Cognition or Communication Ability

Patients with cognitive impairment or an inability to verbalize pain may not be able to indicate the degree of pain, even by using a face scale with pictures of smiling to crying faces. The **Pain Assessment in Advanced Dementia (PAINAD) scale** may be helpful. Careful observation of nonverbal behavior can indicate that the patient is in pain:

- **Respirations**: Patients often have more rapid and labored breathing as pain increases, with short periods of hyperventilation or Cheyne-Stokes respirations.
- **Vocalization**: Patients may remain negative in speech or speak quietly and reluctantly. They may moan or groan. As pain increases, they may call out, moan or groan loudly, or cry.
- **Facial expression**: Patients may appear sad or frightened, may frown or grimace, especially on activities that increase pain.
- **Body language**: Patients may be tense, fidgeting, or pacing, and they may become rigid, clench fists, or lie in fetal position as pain increases. They may become increasingly combative as well.
- **Consolability**: Patients are less distractible or consolable with increased pain.

Wound Etiology

Etiology of Chronic Wounds

Acute wounds heal fairly quickly, moving through stages of healing in a predictable manner; however, chronic wounds behave much differently and outcomes are less predictable. There are a number of factors related to chronic wounds:

- **Wound nature**: Chronic wounds are often related to underlying pathology, such as arterial insufficiency, rather than acute injury. Also, the lack of initial bleeding may impair fibrin production and release of growth factors.
- **Difference in healing**: The initial inflammatory stage of healing is often prolonged because of vascular insufficiency, necrosis, or bacteria.
- **Insufficient growth factors**: Growth factors are necessary to repair tissue, but there are insufficient numbers or they break down quickly, resulting in cellular senescence (inability of cells to proliferate or respond to growth factors).
- **Host factors**: Many factors, such as malnutrition and smoking, may interfere with healing.
- **Denervation**: Lack of adequate innervation impairs the inflammatory response and interferes with healing.

Charcot's Arthropathy

Charcot's arthropathy (Charcot's foot) is the direct result of neuropathy that weakens the muscles of the foot and reduces sensations. The neuropathy weakens the muscles supporting the bones, which in turn become weak and fracture easily. Because of the lack of sensation, the patient may be unaware of the fracture and continue to walk, causing further deformity. The foot becomes inflamed and swollen with increased temperature in foot, but usually there is no pain. In time, the joint dislocation causes the arch to collapse. Treatment includes:

- Compression bandages for 2-3 weeks to reduce edema and inflammation
- Total contact or non-weight-bearing cast applied for up to 9 months
- Gradual weight bearing after skin has resumed normal temperature
- Electrostimulation of the bone may improve healing
- Medications, such as Fosamax and Aredia may be used to decrease bone destruction
- Gradual weight bearing is resumed as foot temperature improves

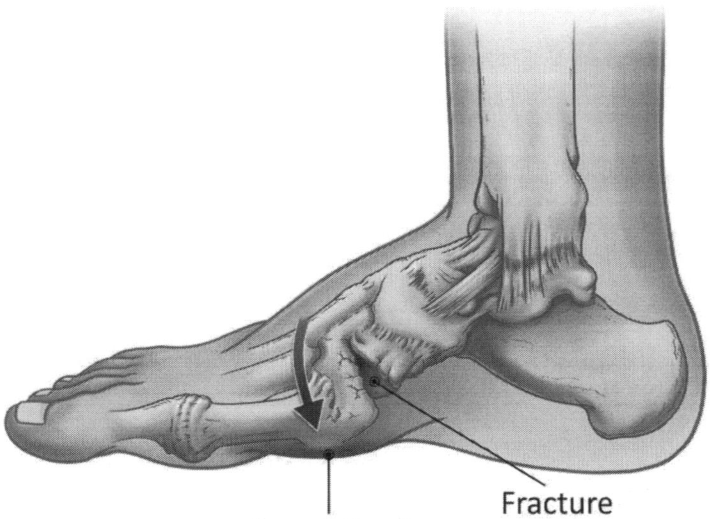

Venous Insufficiency

Venous Ulcers

Venous ulcers were once thought to be caused by venous stasis. Now it is thought that venous hypertension is the cause and the underlying reason that healing doesn't occur. Incompetent valves cause a backup of blood that distends the veins and increases intracapillary pressure. This results in leakage of fluid into the tissues and edema around the ankle areas. Red blood cells leak as well, depositing hemosiderin into the tissues. Hemosiderin is seen as a brownish stain in the lower leg in both Caucasian and black skin. The edematous skin becomes shiny and taut and is extremely itchy. Excoriation and ulceration with infection often occur. The skin may weep or be dry and scaly. Varicose veins and telangiectasia (spider veins) may be seen. The legs feel heavy and ache. A typical venous ulcer has exudate and may have a yellow fibrous film over the wound bed. The shape is irregular and surrounding skin is indurated with a brownish rust color. Scars from previous ulcers are often seen.

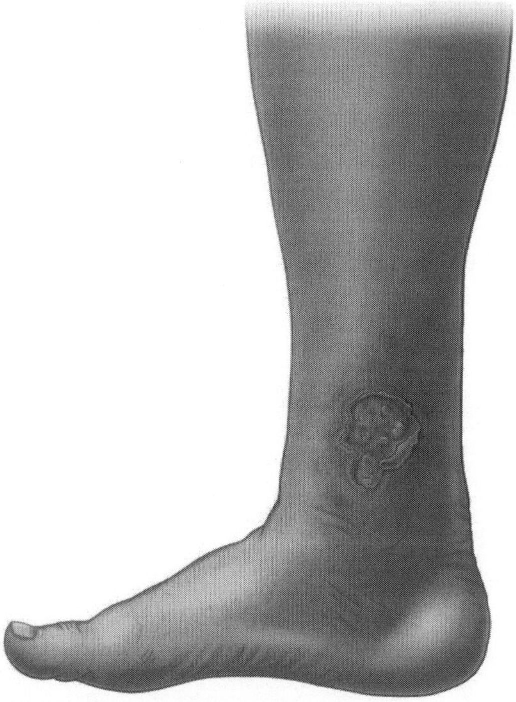

Risk Factors for Chronic Venous Insufficiency

There are a number of risk factors for chronic venous insufficiency (CVI) also known as lower-extremity venous disease (LEVD), primarily those that result in valvular dysfunction or calf-muscle dysfunction:

- **Obesity** with BMI >25 causes patients to be more likely to have pressure on pelvic veins, causing valvular dysfunction.
- **Intravenous drug use** into lower extremities may damage vessels.
- **Thrombosis/leg trauma** may damage vessels and valves.
- **Thrombophlebitis** may cause direct damage to valves.
- **Thrombophilic conditions**, such as protein C deficiency, decrease clotting time of venous blood, increasing risk of thrombosis.
- **Varicose veins** slow venous return.
- **Pregnancy**, especially multiple or close pregnancies increase pressure on pelvic veins.
- **Lack of exercise/sedentary lifestyle** with prolonged periods of sitting result in calf muscle dysfunction.
- **Smoking** causes vascular changes.
- **Age and gender** studies show that older women most commonly develop CVI.
- **Co-morbid conditions**, such as arthritis or those that limit mobility, affect calf-muscle function.

Skin Changes and Abnormalities Related to LEVD

Skin changes and abnormalities, in addition to edema, related to lower-extremity venous disease (LEVD) include:

- **Hemosiderin staining** occurs when hemosiderin, a brownish granular iron-containing pigment resulting from breakdown of hemoglobin, builds up in the interstitial fluid as a result of venous hypertension, causing the erythrocytes to seep into the tissues. As the cells break down, the deposits along with melanin remain in the tissue. This causes a brownish, splotchy discoloration of the skin from the ankle to the anterior tibial area.

- **Lipodermatosclerosis** occurs in the lower leg area as the tissue becomes fibrotic from fibrin and protein (collagen) deposits, causing the skin to feel waxy and the tissue to harden with narrowing of the tissue around the ankle compared to proximal tissue above.
- **Venous (stasis) dermatitis** is inflammation of the epidermis and dermis resulting in scaly, erythematous, crusty, weepy, itchy skin, usually in the lower leg (ankle and tibia). It is progressive with redness and itching appearing before other symptoms.
- **Malleolar flare** is caused by capillaries in a sunburst pattern inferior and distal to the medial malleolus.
- **Atrophie blanche lesions** are smooth white avascular sclerotic skin plaques that occur in about one-third of patients with LEVD. They are usually associated with torturous vessels and hemosiderin staining on the ankles or foot. They may appear similar to scarring from healed ulcers but actually have a high risk for deteriorating into ulcer formation.
- **Varicosities** (varicose veins) are veins where blood has pooled, causing them to become distended, twisted, and palpable, often appearing as blue rope-like vessels on back of the knee and calf or inside of the leg. They are the result of venous reflux and venous hypertension.

Venous Dermatitis

Venous dermatitis appears on the ankles and lower legs and can cause severe itching and pain. Without treatment to control the dermatitis, it may deteriorate, causing ulcers to form, so treatment is needed to alleviate the symptoms:

- Topical antihistamines are used to decrease itching and prevent excoriation from scratching. Low dose topical steroids should be used only for short periods (2 weeks) to reduce inflammation and itching only because of danger of increasing ulceration.
- Compression therapy, usually with compression stockings, is used on affected legs to improve overall venous return.
- Leg elevation when sitting helps to avoid dependency.
- Topical antibiotics, such as bacitracin, should be administered as indicated to reduce danger of infection. Oral antibiotics as indicated for systemic infection.
- Hypoallergenic emollients (without perfume), such as petrolatum jelly, can improve the skin's barrier function and is a preventive measure that should be used when the acute inflammation has subsided.

Arterial Insufficiency

Risk Factors for Lower Extremity Arterial Disease (LEAD)

There are a number of risk factors for lower extremity arterial disease (LEAD):

- **Smoking** is a primary cause of LEAD, with diagnosis of disease 10 years before non-smokers. It increases the rate of atherosclerosis, decreases HDL, increases blood pressure, and decreases clotting time.
- **Obesity** raises blood pressure, decreases HDL in cholesterol while raising cholesterol and triglycerides, and increases risk of circulatory disease, including heart attack.
- **Lack of exercise** decreases pain-free walking distance.
- **Hypertension** correlates with changes in the vessel walls that result in narrowing of blood vessels and decreased circulation.
- **Diabetes mellitus** causes increased plaque formation, decreased clotting time, increased blood viscosity, and hypertrophy of vasculature. Insulin resistance, related to Type II diabetes, increases atherosclerosis. Arterial disease typically progresses faster with diabetes.
- **High blood cholesterol**, especially LDLs, increases atherosclerosis and circulatory impairment.

Subtle Indications of Infection with Arterial Insufficiency

Because of the lack of circulation, the normal signs of inflammation and infection may be evident with arterial insufficiency, so observing for subtle signs of infection is critically important. Prompt identification and treatment is necessary to prevent cellulitis and/or osteomyelitis that may result in amputation. Dry necrotic wounds should be painted with 10% povidone-iodine and covered with dry gauze, but the ulcer and the skin around should be inspected daily. **Indications of infection** include:

- Increased pain in the ischemic limb or ulcer and/or increased edema.
- Increase in necrotic area of ulcer.
- Periwound tissue has fluctuance evident on palpation (soft wave-like texture) that may indicate infection in the tissue.
- Erythema about the perimeter of the wound may be very slight.

At any indication of infection, culture and sensitivities should be done so that appropriate therapy can begin.

Diabetic Wounds

Diabetic Foot Ulcers

Most diabetic ulcers are on the foot, ranging from the toes to the heels. Ulcers may first appear as laceration, blisters, or punctures, and the wound is usually circular with well-defined edges. There is often callus in the periwound tissue. The following are common sites:

- **Toes**: The toes are frequent sites for ulcers because of the potential for trauma. The interphalangeal joints often have limited flexibility that causes pressure and friction. The dorsal toes may have hammertoes from injuries or improperly fitted shoes that are easily injured. Distal toes may suffer injury from poor perfusion, heat, or short footwear.
- **Metatarsal heads** may have poor flexibility, increasing pressure.
- **Bunions** may erode because of deformities or narrow footwear.
- **Midfoot** may suffer injury from trauma or Charcot's fracture.
- **Heels** are susceptible to unrelieved pressure, often related to prolonged periods of bed rest.

Risk Factors

There are a number of risk factors for the development of neuropathic/diabetic ulcers:

- **Sensory loss** can cause sores and ulcers to go undetected in early stages.
- **Vascular insufficiency**, especially peripheral artery disease, occurs four times more frequently in diabetics.
- **Autonomic neuropathy** decreases sweating, leaving feet dry and more prone to cracks and sores.
- Long-term diabetes mellitus with poor glucose control causes severe damage to the circulatory system.
- **Smoking** increases vascular damage and arterial insufficiency.
- **Deformities or lack of mobility** may increase risk of developing ulcers or having ulcers be undetected.
- **Obesity** decreases circulation and interferes with control of diabetes. Between 80% and 90% of diabetics are overweight.
- **Male gender** increases risk.
- **Poor vision** may cause people to overlook dangers or prevent them from examining feet and skin.
- **Age** is associated with an increased danger of ulcers.
- **Ethnic background** can determine genetic risks: Native Americans, Hispanic Americans, African Americans, and Pacific Islanders have higher risk for diabetes, and therefore diabetic neuropathy and ulcers.
- Improperly fitted and supportive footwear can cause ulcerations.

Wound Issues Specific to the Pediatric Population

Pediatric patients, especially infants and young children, have skin that is more fragile and easily injured than that of adults. Incontinence increases risks of tissue breakdown. The incidence of pressure injuries in pediatric and neonatal intensive care units is high with the greatest risk of pressure injuries in children under three being the occiput (because the head is proportionately larger in children). Older children are at increased risk of pressure injuries in the sacral area and heels. Children with intellectual disabilities, spinal cord injuries, and myelomeningocele are especially at risk because of decreased mobility, awareness, and sensation. Risk factors include prolonged immobilization (such as with premature infants), medical equipment/devices that apply pressure to the tissue (such as NG and IV tubing and arm boards). Pressure redistribution devices intended for adults are not always effective with children because of their smaller size and weight, so products intended for pediatric patients should be utilized. Appropriate pain assessment tools, such as NIPS, CHEOPS, and NCCPC, should be utilized as children may express pain differently from adults.

Contact Dermatitis

Contact dermatitis is a localized response to contact with an allergen, resulting in a rash that may blister and itch. Common allergens include poison oak, poison ivy, latex, benzocaine, nickel, and preservatives, but there is a wide range of items, elements, and products to which people may react.

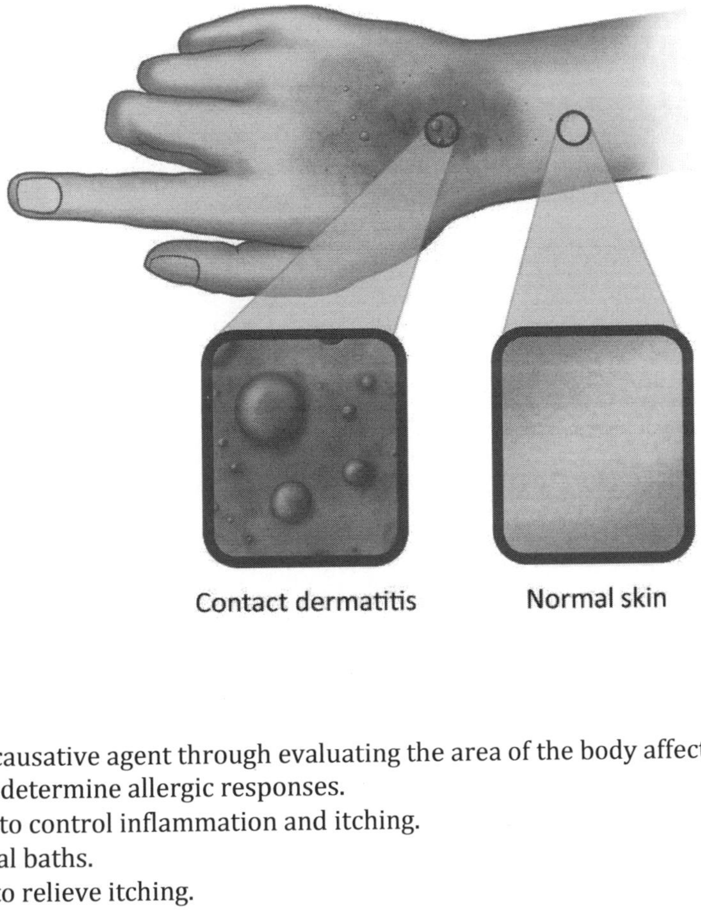

Treatment includes:

- Identifying the causative agent through evaluating the area of the body affected, careful history, or skin patch testing to determine allergic responses.
- Corticosteroids to control inflammation and itching.
- Soothing oatmeal baths.
- Caladryl lotion to relieve itching.
- Antihistamines to reduce allergic response.
- Lesions should be gently cleansed and observed for signs of secondary infection.
- Antibiotics are used only for secondary infections as indicated.
- Rash is usually left open to dry.
- Avoidance of allergen will prevent recurrence.

Candidiasis

Candidiasis, infection of the epidermis with *Candida* spp. (commonly referred to as "yeast" or "thrush"), causes a pustular erythematous papular rash that is commonly scaly, crusty, and macerated with a white cheese-like exudate. It may burn, is usually extremely pruritic, and grows in warm moist areas of the skin, such as under breasts, in abdominal folds, and in the perineal area. Antibiotic use, immunocompromised status, and diabetes mellitus may predispose people to fungal infections, so candidiasis must be differentiated from bacterial infections because antibiotic treatment will worsen the condition. Treatment includes:

- Preventing humid, moist conditions of skin
- Controlling hyperglycemia
- Burow's solution soaks with air drying to relieve itching
- Topical antifungal creams (clotrimazole, nystatin, fluconazole, and ketoconazole) twice daily
- Topical antifungal powders for mild cases
- Oral antifungal medications for severe cases

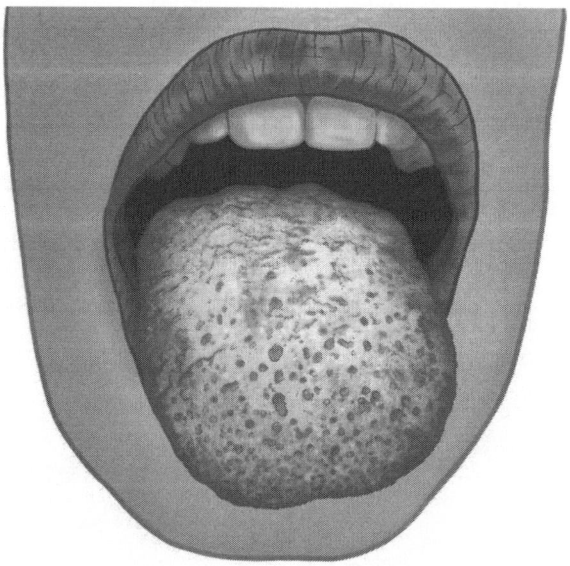

Management of Bacterial Infections

Folliculitis and Impetigo

Folliculitis is a bacterial infection of the hair follicles, often on the face, resulting in pustules, erythema, and crusts that are painful and itchy. Recently, there has been an increase in cases of community-acquired methicillin-resistant *Staphylococcus aureus* folliculitis infections. Folliculitis may occur as a primary or secondary infection and may result from chronic nasal colonization of *MRSA.*

Treatment includes:

- Antibacterial soaps
- Topical or oral antibiotics

Impetigo is a contagious itchy bacterial infection of the skin, commonly on the face or hands, causing clusters of blisters or sores, especially in children. Group A *Streptococcus* usually causes small blisters that crust over. *Staphylococcus aureus* usually causes larger blisters that may be bullous and cause lesions 2-8cm in size that persist for months. Treatment includes:

- Avoid itching
- Gently cleanse area with soap and water
- Topical Bactroban 3 times daily until healed

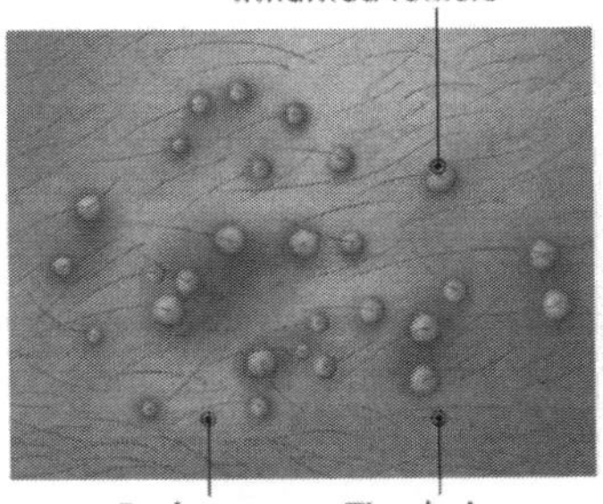

Folliculitis

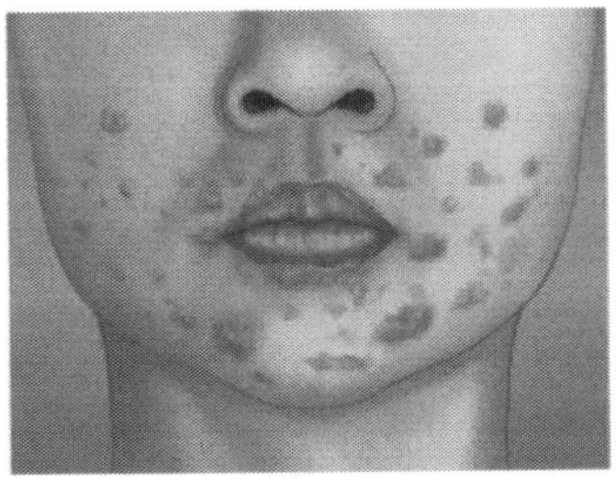

Impetigo

Staphylococcal Scalded Skin Syndrome

Staphylococcal scalded skin syndrome (SSSS) is a superficial partial-thickness infection of the skin caused by toxins produced by a localized *Staphylococcus aureus* infection, resulting in generalized erythema followed in 24-48 hours by blisters that rupture and peel off, leaving large areas of superficial necrosis and denuded skin, giving the skin a burned or "scalded" appearance. It is most common in neonates and children under 5 but can affect adults who are immunocompromised or in renal failure. Pain is usually mild unless the infection is very widespread. Treatment includes:

- IV antibiotics (such as flucloxacillin) are usually needed initially, followed by a course of oral antibiotics.
- Maintenance of fluids and electrolytes.
- Debridement of skin.
- Moisture-retentive dressings, such as foam dressings, sheet hydrogels, and alginates, avoiding adhesives.
- Excessive tissue loss may be treated the same as partial-thickness burns.

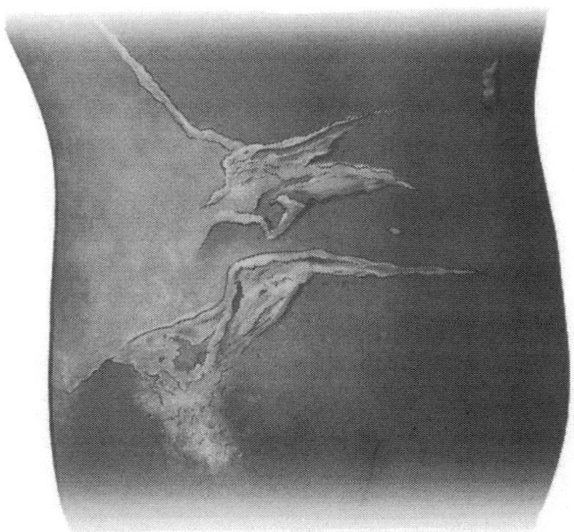

Erysipelas

Erysipelas is a superficial bacterial infection, primarily of the face or legs, involving the cutaneous lymphatic system and invading the skin in areas of trauma. Facial erysipelas is usually caused by group A *Streptococcus* following a nasopharyngeal infection. Infections on the legs are more often related to non-group A *Streptococcus.* The infection spreads rapidly with streaking and clearly demarcated erythema and cellulitis. Local lymph nodes become inflamed, sometimes resulting in lymphedema because of damage to lymph nodes. Erysipelas most commonly affects children and the elderly. Treatment includes:

- Bed rest with elevation of affected limb and warm saline packs to improve circulation.
- Oral antibiotic (usually penicillin G and penicillin VK). IV antibiotics may be indicated for severe cases.
- Hospitalization is recommended for severe cases or those who are very young, elderly, or immunocompromised.
- Analgesics to control pain.

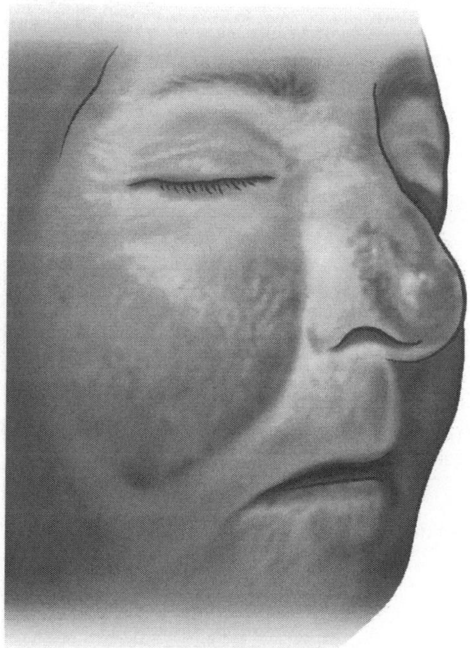

Toxic Shock Syndrome

Toxic shock syndrome (TSS) is an acute, severe life-threatening bacterial infection that causes a systemic infection with high fever, hypotension, myalgia, diarrhea, and widespread erythematous rash that has the appearance of bad sunburn, with subsequent desquamation (peeling). The original causative agent was *Staphylococcus aureus* and infections were related to the use of tampons, but the infection can occur with wounds or surgical sites where the bacteria can find entry. There are now 2 forms: *Staphylococcus aureus* (TSS) and *Streptococcal* toxic shock syndrome (STSS). *STSS* occurs secondary to an infection in the body, often an infected wound, causing severe hypotension, dyspnea, tachycardia, liver and kidney failure, and a splotchy rash that may peel. Treatment includes:

- Hospitalization for aggressive antibiotic therapy
- Intravenous fluids to treat hypotension
- Topical non-adhesive, non-occlusive dressings with absorbent materials as indicated

Herpes Zoster

Herpes zoster ("shingles") is caused by varicella zoster virus retained in the nerve cells after childhood chickenpox. The virus remains dormant until it is reactivated, often in older adults who are immunocompromised. Initial symptoms include pain (often severe burning) and redness. Painful blistering lesions then occur along sensory nerves, usually in a line from the spine around to the chest, although sometimes the head and face are involved. Facial nerve involvement can cause loss of taste and hearing. Eye involvement can cause blindness. The lesions eventually crust over and heal in 2-4 weeks, although some have persistent post-herpetic neuralgia for 6-12 months or longer. The lesions are contagious to those who contact them and have not been immunized or had chickenpox.

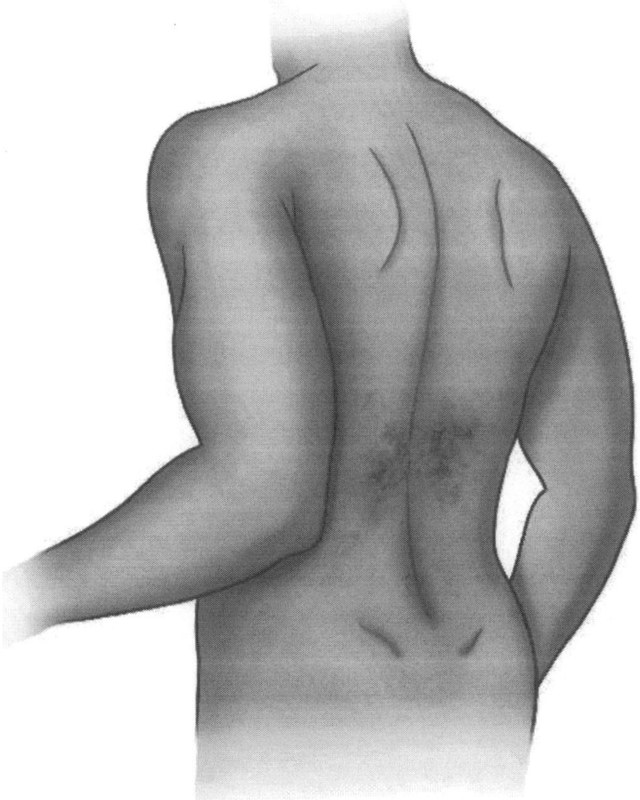

Necrotizing Fasciitis

Necrotizing fasciitis is a rapidly spreading infection of the soft tissues involving extensive necrosis of the fascia and subcutaneous tissue as well as destruction of the vasculature with thrombosis. It most often occurs in the extremities after a minor infection. The most common organisms are group A β-hemolytic *Streptococci*, but there may be polymicrobial infections or other causative agents. It may result from surgical procedures, including cardiac catheterization. The infection begins with pain, edema, fever, toxemia, and cellulitis that spreads rapidly, becoming increasingly cyanotic as tissue and perfusion is impaired. Bullae form and progress to necrosis, gangrene, and sepsis within 3-5 days. Mortality rates are 25%. Treatment includes:

- Aggressive extensive surgical debridement of all non-viable tissue. Repeat surgical debridement may be necessary.
- Antibiotic therapy.
- Wound care as indicated by the extent of the wound with careful monitoring to determine if the wound is deteriorating.
- IV immunoglobulin may be used.

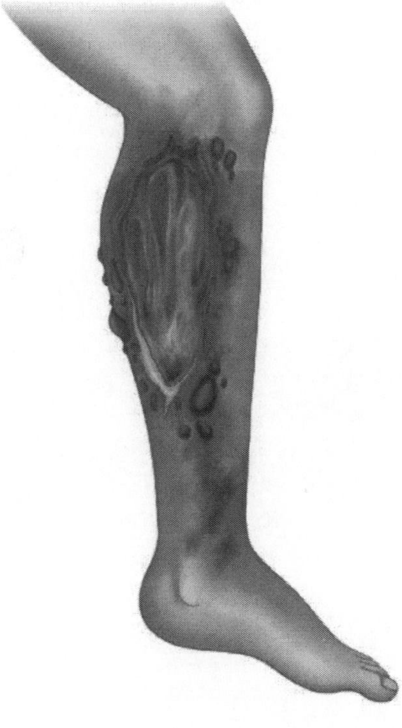

Pemphigus Vulgaris

Pemphigus vulgaris (PV), an autoimmune disorder causing blistering of both the skin and the mucous membranes (presenting symptoms in 50-70% of patients), creates burn-like wounds, which may heal slowly or not at all, often starting in the mouth and genital areas. Untreated the disorder can lead to death. Blisters on skin rupture, causing ulcerations, and those in folds may develop hypergranulation and crusting. Treatment includes:

- Corticosteroids (Prednisone) and immunosuppressive drugs (Imuran).
- Nutritional assessment: vitamin D and calcium supplement may be needed.
- Careful observation for secondary infections.
- Protective clothing and minimize trauma to skin.
- Rituxan, a drug used for lymphoma and leukemia, has helped patients go into remission when used with other drugs.
- Sheets should be kept clean and dry at all times, and changed immediately when soiled.
- Good oral care with soft toothbrush.
- Plasmapheresis with plasma removed to reduce antibodies and donated plasma infused.
- Potassium permanganate lotion bath (1:10000) and chlorhexidine tulle gauze dressing of the denuded areas.

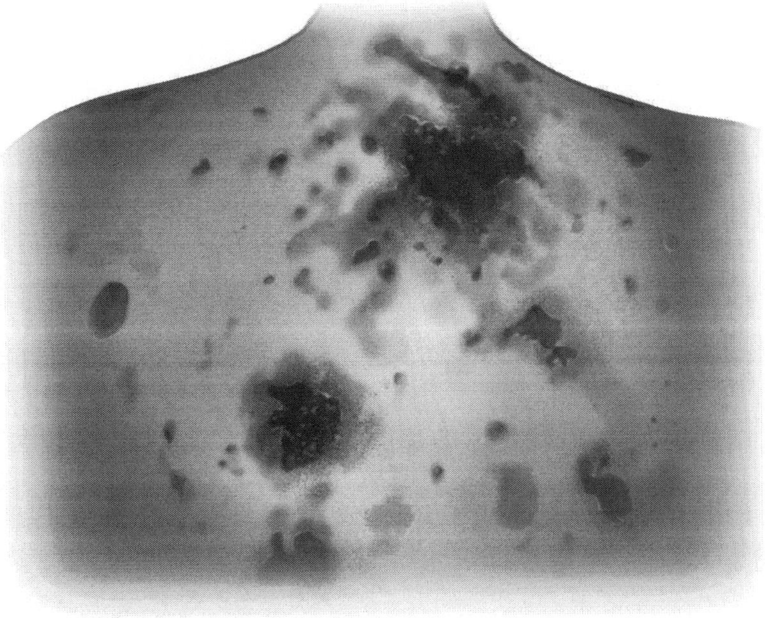

Fungating Neoplastic Wounds

Fungating neoplastic wounds occur in up to 10% of those with metastasis, especially involving oral or breast cancer. Fungating wounds are ulcerating with necrosis and slough and may have a foul odor and small to copious amount of drainage. Infection is common and the periwound tissue may become inflamed, macerated, or tender. The prognosis is very poor and treatment may be primarily palliative, depending upon the condition of the patient:

- **Control bleeding**: The ulcers bleed as the vasculature erodes, so hemostatic dressings (Gel foam, alginates) and cauterization with silver nitrate may be necessary. Use non-adherent dressings or long-term dressings to reduce trauma.
- **Manage exudate**: Foam, alginate, or hydrofiber dressings or wound pouch as indicated.
- **Control odor**: Use of charcoal dressing or Chloromycetin solution.
- **Protect periwound tissue**: Skin sealants, barrier ointments, and hydrocolloid waters to anchor tape.
- **Cleanse wound**: Use ionic cleansers or antiseptics.
- **Control pain**: Analgesia as indicated.

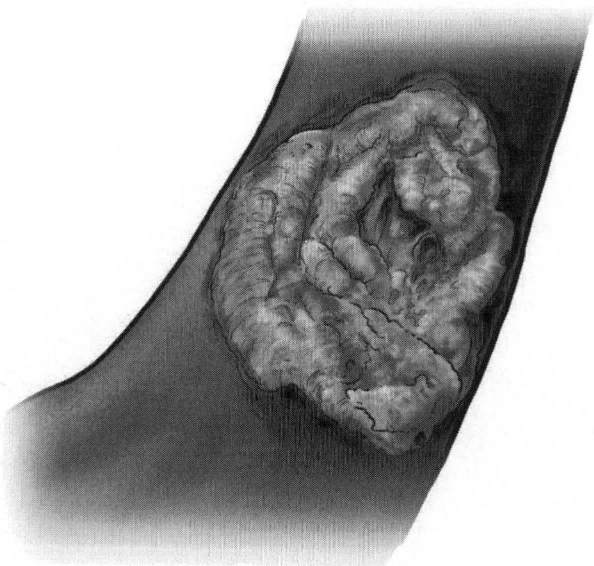

CALCIPHYLAXIS

Calciphylaxis is a rare fatal disease related to end-stage renal disease and uremia, resulting in vascular calcification of cutaneous blood vessels and necrotic lesions with typical violet discoloration. Mortality rates range from 60-80%, usually caused by sepsis. Patients present with painful discolored lesions that progress to nodules and ulcerations that become infected and gangrenous. Lesions are most common in areas with accumulation of fatty tissue. Blood flow distal to the ulcerations is usually intact. The etiology is unclear, but it is associated with hypercalcemia, hyperphosphatemia, and hyperparathyroidism. Treatment is often palliative as there is no successful standardized approach, although the disorder frequently results in amputation of the affected limb.

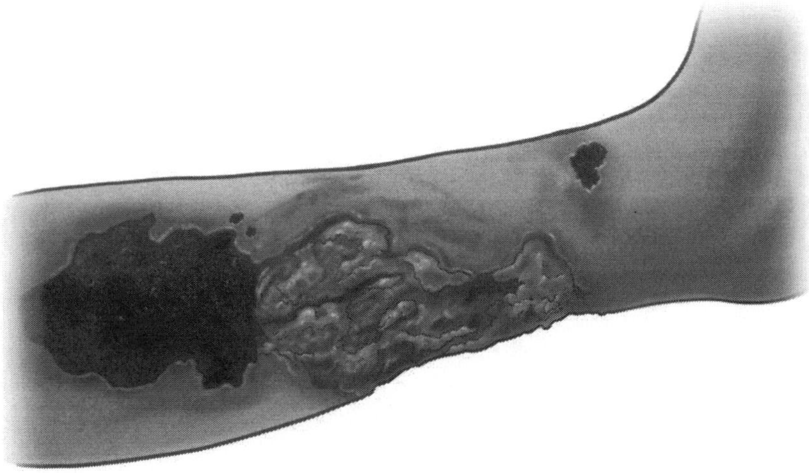

Treatment includes:

- Control of calcium and phosphorus levels
- Intravenous sodium thiosulfate to reduce calcium deposits
- Surgical or medical treatment of hyperparathyroidism
- Antibiotics as indicated for wound infections
- Aggressive debridement with absorbent moisture-retentive dressings
- Analgesia as indicated

Pyoderma Granulosum

Pyoderma granulosum is a painful ulcerative condition of the skin that is often associated with underlying systemic diseases (such as inflammatory bowel disease) and dysregulation of immunity involving neutrophils. There are two types:

- **Classical**: Deep ulcerations with border overhanging wound bed, most common on the legs but may be around stomas.
- **Atypical**: Vesiculopustular draining lesions, usually on the tops of the hands, the forearms, or face.

Treatment includes:

- Topical and systemic corticosteroids and systemic immunosuppressive drugs
- Local wound care and dressings as indicated for the type and degree of wound, includes moisture-retentive non-adherent dressings
- Autolysis is only debridement because of danger of extending the disease
- Topical antibiotics may be necessary to control infection
- Treating the underlying systemic cause, such as colectomy for ulcerative colitis, may reduce symptoms
- Surgical treatment of lesions is usually avoided

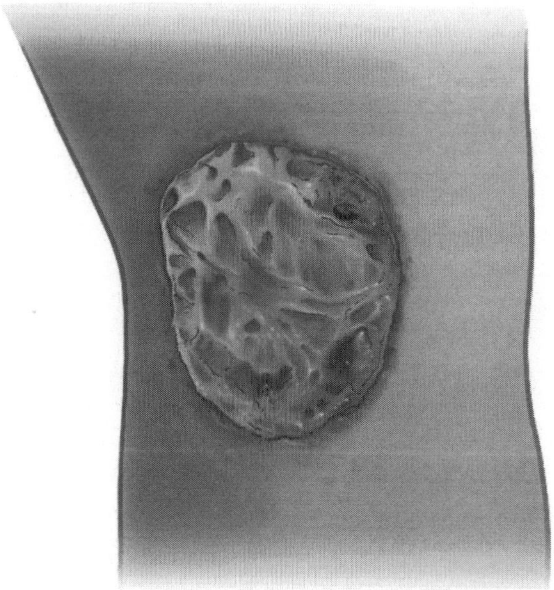

Epidermolysis Bullosa

Epidermolysis bullosa (EB) comprises a group of inherited and non-inherited bullous (blistering) disorders of different levels of the epithelial tissue, with even mild mechanical trauma resulting in blistering. Symptoms vary widely and may range from slight seasonal blistering to life-threatening erosions of skin. It may affect internal epithelial tissue in mucous membranes and organs as well as the external dermal layers. There are different **categories** of EB:

- **Simplex (EBS)**: Intraepidermal lesions.
- **Junctional (JEB)**: Blistering at lamina lucida (between epidermis and basement membrane).
- **Recessive dystrophic (RDEB)**: Separation at basement membrane. Excessive scarring and blistering from slight mechanical trauma, leading to hemorrhage and ulceration. Predisposes to squamous cell carcinoma.
- **Dominant dystrophic (DDEB)**: Blisters below basement membrane with scarring, less severe than RDEB.

Treatment includes:

- Nutritional assessment and supplements as needed
- Topical antibiotics or silver-impregnated dressings for infection
- Protection to avoid trauma
- Fenestrated non-adherent dressings, secured with stockinet, roll gauze, or tubular gauze

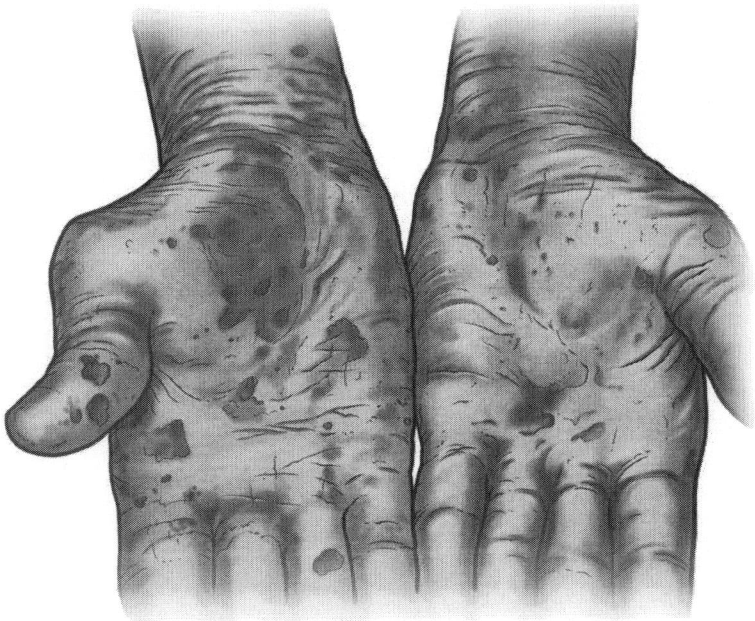

Vasculitis

Vasculitis comprises a large number of disorders that result in inflammation of veins, arteries, and capillaries, causing changes in vessel walls. Symptoms vary widely, but frequently include fever, general malaise, myalgia, loss of appetite, and skin lesions. Skin lesions may range from macular rashes to large necrotic ulcerations. Lesions are commonly on the lower extremities and may be confused with venous lesions. Disorders that may cause vasculitis with hemorrhagic rash or ulcerations include Behcet's syndrome, Henoch-Schönlein purpura, rheumatoid vasculitis, systemic lupus erythematosus, polyarteritis nodosa, and Wegener's granulomatosis.

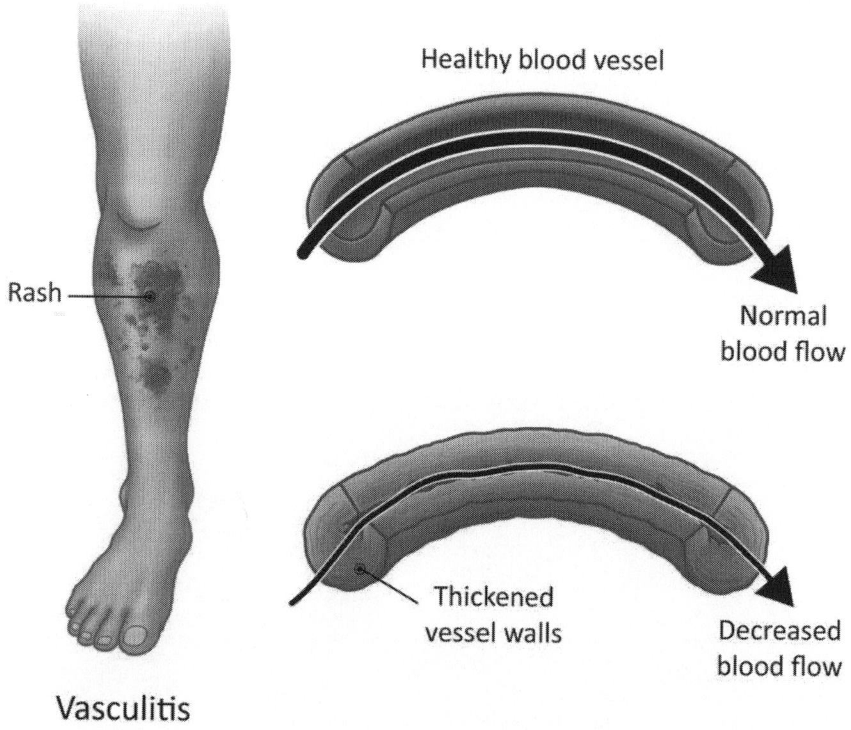

Treatment includes:

- Medical control of underlying disease process
- Systemic corticosteroids, antihistamines, and immunosuppressants
- Debridement of necrosis
- Observation for infection and treatment with topical or systemic antibiotics as indicated
- Moisture retentive dressings with absorptive material if needed for exudate
- Skin sealants or barriers to protect periwound tissue from exudate
- Monitor nutrition and provide supplements as needed

Toxic Epidermal Necrolysis

Toxic epidermal necrolysis is a rare life-threatening condition of the epidermis caused by drug reactions to 3 types of drugs: antibiotics (sulfonamides, allopurinol, and ampicillin), anticonvulsants (phenytoin, carbamazepine, and phenobarbital), and analgesics (acetaminophen and NSAIDS). An initial maculopapular rash gives way to erythema and painful skin that sloughs with the slightest pressure, leaving >10% of the body denuded of epidermis. The skin, mucous membranes, eyes, and respiratory tract may be involved with mortality rates of 30-40%. Treatment includes:

- Surgical debridement of sloughing skin with saline-moistened cloth
- Porcine xenografts stapled into place
- Patient placed in air-fluidized bed in burn unit
- Fluid and electrolytes monitored and replaced
- NG feedings
- Systemic antibiotics and cessation of any corticosteroids
- Pain control with opioids
- Pulmonary and ophthalmic care
- Grafts trimmed as they desiccate and wounds heal

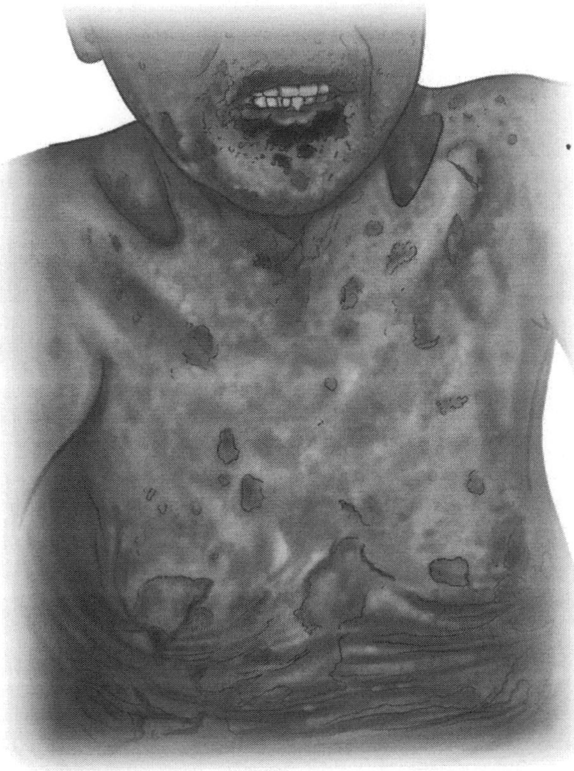

Graft-Versus-Host Disease

Graft-versus-host disease (GVHD) is caused by a severe host reaction to bone marrow or stem cell transplantation. Acute GVHD occurs within 100 days after surgery, and chronic GVHD occurs after 100 days. The skin, liver (causing jaundice and pruritus), and large and small intestines (causing bleeding and diarrhea) may all be involved. A maculopapular (red to violet) rash usually begins on the hands, plantar area of the feet, face, and upper trunk, then spreads and may results in desquamation and formation of bullae. The disease is staged 1-4 depending on severity.

Treatment includes:

- Colony-stimulating factor (CSF) for 6 months and other appropriate immunosuppressive therapy.
- Topical corticosteroids may be used.
- Careful observation and cleansing of skin for signs of infection.
- Severe denudement requires debridement and transfer to the burn unit for treatment appropriate to the condition to prevent further deterioration.
- Adhesive occlusive dressings should be avoided.

Classification of Burns

Burn injuries may be chemical, electrical, or thermal and are assessed by the area affected, percentage of the body burned, and the depth of the burn, as follows:

- **First-degree burns** are superficial and affect the epidermis, causing erythema and pain.
- **Second-degree burns** extend through the dermis (partial thickness), resulting in blistering and sloughing of the epidermis and severe pain.
- **Third-degree burns** affect the underlying tissue, including the vasculature, muscles, and nerves (full thickness). Depending on the extent of the nerve damage, third-degree burns may present with less pain.

Burns are **classified** according to the American Burn Association's criteria as follows:

- **Minor**: <10% body surface area (BSA) in adults or <5% in children and elderly, or 2% BSA with third-degree burns without serious risk to the face, hands, feet, or perineum.
- **Moderate**: 10–20% BSA combined second- and third-degree burns in adults or 5-10% in children or elderly, or 2-5% third-degree burns without serious risk to the face, hands, feet, or perineum.
- **Major**: >20% BSA in adults or >10% in children/elderly; >5% third-degree burns; any burns that are to the face, hands, feet, or perineum and will result in functional/cosmetic defect; or burns with inhalation or other major trauma.

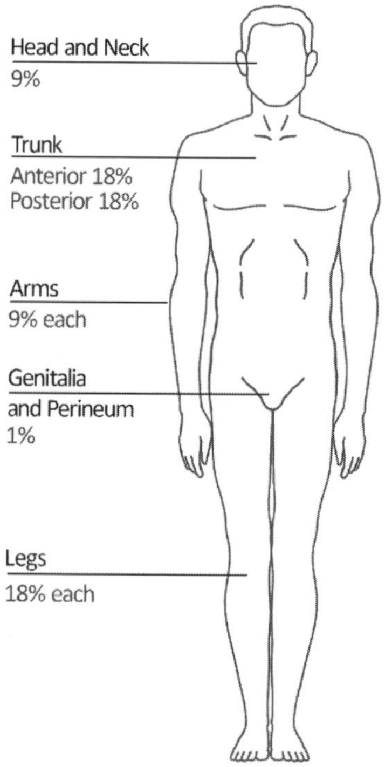

Rule of Nines

The Rule of Nines is helpful when assessing burn patients to determine if IV fluids (needed if ≥10% total BSA) or transfer to a burn unit is necessary (needed if >20% total BSA, 2nd degree >10% total BSA, 3rd degree >5% total BSA).

Note that the percentage calculations are modified for infants and children under 10 years old because of their larger head and smaller body size. The head is assigned 18%, and the legs are given 13.5% each.

Review Video: Rule of Nines
Visit mometrix.com/academy and enter code: 846800

Complications Associated with Burn Injuries

Burn injuries begin with the skin but can affect all organs and body systems, especially with a major burn. Complications include the following:

- **Cardiovascular**: Cardiac output may fall by 50% as capillary permeability increases with vasodilation and fluid leaks from the tissues, resulting in hypovolemia and hypothermia. Vasoconstriction occurs as a compensatory mechanism, but it may impair circulation and result in further hypoxia.
- **Pulmonary**: Injury may result from smoke inhalation or (rarely) aspiration of hot liquid. Pulmonary injury is a leading cause of death from burns and is classified according to the degree of damage as follows:
    - **First**: Singed eyebrows and nasal hairs with possible soot in airways and slight edema, increasing hypoxia.
    - **Second**: Stridor, dyspnea, and tachypnea with edema and erythema of the upper airway, including the area of the vocal cords and epiglottis, resulting in severe hypoxia, sometimes with rapid onset.
- **Infection**: Open wounds are vulnerable to infection.
- **Circumferential burns**: Swelling beneath eschar can create a tourniquet effect, impairing distal circulation.

Electrical Burns

Electricity injures the skin by heating tissues and destroying cellular membranes:

- **Flash burns** look the same as a thermal burn and any hair in the area will be singed. This is the type of burn that usually occurs when a person is struck by lightning. There may be entry and exit burns.
- **Arc burns,** in which the patient is part of a circuit of electricity (≤4000 °C) arcing through the air, have a dry parchment-like center with a surrounding circle of congestion.
- **Contact burns** may show a branding the size of the object touched. Hair is not usually burned in this case.

High-voltage burns of the extremities may require a fasciotomy to save the limb. Care at a specialized burn center is needed for those with moderate to severe burns or for those with electrical burns around the mouth. Disfigurement may be severe when nerves and muscles are destroyed.

Lightning Burns and Injuries

Lightning burns and injuries may occur with a direct strike (≤5%), side splash from a strike nearby, contact voltage when touching an item that has been struck, ground current (from a more distant strike), and blunt trauma from being too close to a strike (which often results in the patient being thrown). Symptoms may vary, but they can include external burns (Lichtenberg figures) in a fernlike pattern, acute pain, fixed and dilated pupils (temporary), eye injuries, confusion, headache, hearing loss, perforated eardrum, hypotension, paralysis/paresis, spinal cord injury, altered mental status, brain injury, fractures, and cardiac arrest. Patients may be responsive initially but lapse into unconsciousness as cerebral edema increases, resulting in secondary respiratory and/or cardiac arrest. Burns are usually mild because of the brief contact.

Management of Burn Injuries

Management of burn injuries must include both wound care and systemic care. Treatment includes establishment of airway, treatment for inhalation injury, and intravenous fluids and electrolytes, based on weight and extent of burn.

$$\text{Parkland formula: } 4\text{ mL/kg/day} \times \text{BSA\%}$$

The type of wound treatment depends upon the **severity** of the burn:

- **First-degree**: Superficial and affects the epidermis. Usually, only emollients are needed and symptoms recede within 3-4 days, usually with peeling skin.
- **Second-degree**: Superficial partial-thickness. The skin blisters and sloughs off, denuding the area. These burns may be very painful. Silvadene or other silver preparations are commonly applied to the burns in the initial stages. The skin is debrided and covered with dressings, which are changed every 1-3 days. Healing usually occurs within 2 weeks.
- **Third-degree**: Deep partial-thickness through the epidermis and the dermis. The wounds are painful and may be wet or dry and nonblanchable. The wound requires debridement and grafting as they rarely heal on their own.
- **Fourth-degree**: Full-thickness and may extend through muscle, vessels, and nerves. Third-degree burns require extensive debridement, grafting to prevent massive protein/fluid loss and infection, and application of topical antibiotics and compression dressings.

Skin Damage Caused by Radiation Treatment

Skin damage/burns caused by radiation treatment vary widely depending upon the dose, duration, fraction-size, treatment area, and type of equipment as well as the condition of the patient. Acute radiation dermatitis usually occurs when radiation is higher than 10 Gy. Patients vary in the progression of symptoms. There may be an initial inflammatory response in the tissue, with increased perfusion and WBCs to the area.

Staging of Skin Damage

Acute skin damage begins within 2-3 weeks of exposure to radiation with changes that are reversible. Because the cells in the skin are constantly going through mitotic division, they are vulnerable to the effects of irradiation. Most reactions subside 1-3 months after therapy ends. Damage is staged according to the type and degree of reaction, and staging determines treatment:

- **Stage I**: Slight edema and inflammation with erythema that may result in burning, itching, and discomfort, caused by dilation and increased permeability of capillaries.
- **Stage II**: Dry, itching, scaly skin with partial sloughing of epidermis, caused by inability of basal epidermal cells to adequately replace surface cells and decreased functioning of skin glands.
- **Stage III**: Moist blistering skin with loss of epidermal tissue, serous drainage, and increased pain with exposure of nerves, caused by continued deterioration of skin.
- **Stage IV**: Loss of body hair and sweat gland suppression resulting in permanent hair loss, atrophy, pigment changes, and ulcerations, caused by accumulation of radiation in the tissues.

Treatment for Radiation Damage

Management of tissue damage related to irradiation focuses on treating damage and preventing deterioration in order to relieve discomfort and promote healing. Patients must be educated about the need for skin care during therapy:

- **Protect skin** by maintaining cleanliness, avoiding irritants, using electric razors, protecting the skin from sunlight and extremes of heat and cold, applying appropriate emollients, using mild soaps, and wearing loose, protective clothing.
- **Relieve discomfort** by using cornstarch or powders (NOT talcum) in dry areas, applying topical corticosteroids sparingly to reduce itching.
- **Treat open areas** by using saline compresses, Sitz baths, and semi-occlusive dressings as indicated to protect nerve endings. Prevent damage to wounds by using non-adherent dressings and securing them with mesh or stockinet instead of tape. Culture wounds and treat bacterial or fungal infections as indicated. Use dressings appropriate for the amount and type of exudate to prevent further skin damage or irritation of periwound skin.

Assessment of Pressure Injuries

When assessing a tissue injury, it is necessary to determine whether it is a pressure injury or non-pressure injury because the treatment protocol may vary depending upon whether the injury is caused by pressure, venous or arterial insufficiency, or neuropathic disorders. The clinical basis for this determination should be clearly outlined.

- The pressure injury should be classified according to the stage and the characteristics, including size (length, width, and depth).
- Pain associated with the pressure injury should be described.
- Photographs should be taken if a protocol is in place.
- Pressure injuries should be monitored daily and any changes carefully documented.
- The injury should be evaluated for signs of infection.

It is important to differentiate between colonization, which is very common, and infection, which usually presents with symptoms such as periwound erythema, induration, and increased pain as well as delayed healing of the wound. Wound culture and blood tests should be done if there are indications of infection. Treatment should be determined according to the characteristics of the wound.

Causes of Pressure Injuries

Pressure Intensity, Pressure Duration, and Tissue Tolerance

Pressure injuries are caused primarily by pressure, but there are numerous additional considerations:

- **Pressure intensity***:* Capillary closing pressure (10–32 mmHg) is the minimal pressure needed to collapse capillaries, reducing tissue perfusion. This pressure can be easily exceeded in the sitting or supine position if weight is not shifted.
- **Duration of pressure**: Low pressure for long periods and high pressure for short periods can both result in pressure injuries.
- **Tissue tolerance***:* The tissue tolerance is the ability of the skin to tolerate and redistribute pressure, preventing anoxia. Both extrinsic and intrinsic factors can affect tissue tolerance. Extrinsic factors include shear (the skin stays in place but the underlying tissue slides), friction (moving the skin against bedding or other objects), and moisture. Intrinsic factors include poor nutrition, advanced age, low blood pressure, stress, smoking, and low body temperature.

Shear and Friction

Shear occurs when the skin stays in place and the underlying tissue in the deep fascia over the bony prominences stretches and slides, damaging vessels and tissue and often resulting in undermining. Shear is one of the most common causes of pressure injuries, which are often described as pressure ulcers but are technically somewhat different, although the effects of shearing are often combined with pressure. The most common cause of shear is elevation of the head of the bed over 30°. Friction against the sheets holds the skin in place while the body slides down the bed, resulting in pressure and damage in the sacrococcygeal area. The underlying vessels are damaged and thrombosed, leading to undermining and deep ulceration.

Friction is a significant cause of pressure injuries because it acts with gravity to cause shear. Friction by itself results only in damage to the epidermis and dermis, such as abrasions or denudement referred to as "sheet burn." Friction and pressure can combine, however, to form tissue injury.

Measures to Control Shear and Friction

Because **shear** and **friction** are primary factors in the development of pressure injuries, measures to reduce them are essential:

- The head of the bed should never be elevated more than 30°; however, bed-bound patients may not be able to feed themselves at this angle. If the bed is elevated higher, the patient should be carefully positioned, using a pull sheet or overhead trapeze to make sure the patient is at the right position. The bed should be lowered as soon as possible.

Note: Elevating the foot of the bed to prevent sliding and shear simply increases pressure to the sacrococcygeal area, solving one problem by creating another.

- Making sure that the skin is dry; using fine cornstarch-based powders may help prevent the skin from "sticking" to the sheets.
- Pull sheets or mechanical lifting devices should be used to lift, move, or transfer the patient.
- Medical treatments may reduce restlessness.
- Heel and elbow protectors provide protection.

Management of Pressure Injuries

Measures to Promote Mobility

Mobility is a problem for many patients with pressure injuries because their restricted mobility is often the cause of the injury in the first place. However, promoting mobility to the extent possible improves circulation, aids healing, and decreases risk of developing further pressure injury:

- Bed-bound patients must be repositioned on a scheduled basis and should receive passive ROM exercises and active bed exercises if tolerated daily. The patient's head should be elevated only to 30° for short periods of time.
- Patients with limited mobility should be evaluated by physical and occupational therapists in order to develop an individualized plan for activities. Patients may need assistive devices, such as walkers, canes, or wheelchairs. Because the wound must be protected without compromise to circulation, the amount and type of mobility or exercises must be designed with respect to the area and stage of the pressure injury as well as underlying pathology or co-morbid conditions.

Measures to Control Fecal Incontinence

Control of fecal incontinence is necessary to prevent deterioration of tissue that can increase the risk of pressure injuries and to prevent contamination of existing pressure injuries:

- Assess incontinence to determine cause and whether it is temporary, related to health problems, or chronic.
- Determine the type of incontinence:
    - Passive, in which the person is unaware.
    - Urge, which is the inability to retain stool.
    - Seepage, after a bowel movement or around a blockage.
- Use medications as indicated to control diarrhea or constipation.
- Place on a bowel-training regimen with scheduled bowel movements, using suppositories, stool softeners, and bulk formers as indicated, according to cause of incontinence. Use skin moisture barriers and absorbent pads or adult briefs as needed.
- Modify diet as needed with foods to control diarrhea or constipation.
- Ensure adequate fluid intake.
- Consider fecal pouches or fecal containment devices if incontinence cannot be otherwise controlled.

Measures to Control Urinary Incontinence

Control of urinary incontinence is necessary to prevent deterioration of the tissue that can increase the risk of pressure injuries:

- Assess incontinence to determine cause and whether it is temporary, related to health problems, or chronic.
- A temporary Foley catheter may be used in some cases while tissue heals, but long-term use is contraindicated because of the danger of infections.
- Medications may be indicated to treat urinary infections or frequency. Scheduled toileting with reinforcement may help to decrease incidence.
- Use absorbent pads or adult briefs that wick liquid away from the body, and establish a regular schedule for changing.
- Cleanse soiled skin with no-rinse wipes, as they are less drying to skin than soap and water.
- Use skin moisture barrier ointments to protect skin from urine.
- Use protective and support devices as needed.
- Avoid positioning on existing pressure injuries.

Factors Influencing the Healing of Surgical Wounds

There are a number of **factors that affect surgical wound healing**:

- Preoperative showering and skin preparation without shaving decreases incidence of infection.
- Patient condition prior to surgery, type of illness, and the procedure performed all affect healing.
- Breaks in sterile procedure, contamination of the wound by the GI tract, or encountering inflammation or necrotic tissues during the course of the surgery creates a "dirty" wound that has a greater chance of infection.
- Longer procedures increase infection risk.
- The amount of mechanical stress on tissues during the surgery affects inflammation.
- The wound must have a proper blood supply and be able to be closed without causing tension of the tissues.

Topical Therapy for Surgical Wounds

Topical therapy for surgical wounds is generally conservative, observing for signs of healing and infection. The standard use of antimicrobials and antiseptics is generally not indicated because of the danger of resistance and the cytotoxic properties of some that delay healing. Therapy includes:

- Initial dressing to provide protection, to absorb any exudate, and to provide thermal insulation to promote healing. Dressings should be lightly applied in order to prevent compression that may impede perfusion to the wound. These may be left in place for 48-72 hours to allow the wound to begin to seal.
- If there are signs of local infection, a topical antimicrobial (such as Neosporin) or antiseptic (such as povidone iodine) may be applied to the surgical incision site.
- Depending upon the site of the incision, after the initial healing has taken place, the wound may be left uncovered or a soft dressing may be kept in place to prevent local irritation.

Wound Dehiscence

Wound sutures should be long lasting, at times permanent, as opposed to absorbable. They should be placed 1 cm from the wound edge and 1 cm apart. If sutures are too thin, they may stretch, break, or cut through tissues. Knots may become undone if there are too few sutures to hold tissues together adequately when the wound is under tension due to obesity or movement. Suture problems can cause wound dehiscence to occur. Wound dehiscence occurs more often in those older than 65. Other factors include obesity, cancer, emergency surgery situations, steroid use, hypoalbuminemia, and hypovolemia. Wound infections or intra-abdominal sepsis also predisposes the wound to dehiscence. Coughing, vomiting, and ascites put strain on the incision. The first indication of dehiscence is leakage of serosanguineous fluid. Evisceration can occur suddenly or gradually as the incision opens. The patient is taken to surgery and any necrotic tissues are removed to allow the wound to be resutured through healthy tissues. Hernias often form in these scars.

Keloid and Hypertrophic Scars

Keloid scars are thick, rope-like, and extend over the borders of the wound, rarely regressing with healing. Keloids occur more frequently in African Americans and Asians. They occur due to excess collagen deposition, causing increased growth. Normal collagen degradation that occurs in wound remodeling is overtaken by the rate of deposition. Keloids respond to cutting or abrasion by growing even bigger. They are most common on the upper back, chest, earlobes, and deltoids. Keloids may be painful or itch. The tendency to form keloid scars should be assessed when treating a patient's wound so that precautions may be taken in the early stages of wound healing to try to prevent keloid formation.

Hypertrophic scars are also thick but they stay within the borders of the wound and occur most often over joints where there was tension on the wound. They may regress in time. They can also itch, cause pain, and decrease functional movement if they contract.

Factors to Consider About Traumatic Wounds

There are many types of traumatic wounds: slashes, incisions, crush injuries, degloving, and penetrating. However, they hold the following elements in common:

- Traumatic wounds may not only have tissue trauma but also trauma to blood vessels, nerves, tendons, muscles, and bone.
- There may be extensive bleeding that must be stopped.
- The wound may be contaminated with bacteria, dirt, or foreign bodies that must be removed with irrigation or exploration. Wounds that are contaminated or missing significant tissue must remain open to heal by secondary intention.
- There may be nonviable tissue that must be removed, requiring skin grafts to cover the underlying tissue.
- Wounds involving joint capsules are at risk for septic arthritis, and those of the extremities may be at risk for compartment syndrome, requiring a fasciotomy to save the limb from ischemia due to edema.

Treatment of Traumatic Bite Wounds

Animal Bites

There is no one topical therapy for traumatic wounds because they vary so widely in the type and degree of injury. A scrape on the knee is treated very differently from a car accident that involves massive tissue injury or tissue loss. Animal bites, including human, are frequent causes of traumatic injury. Treatment includes:

- Cleanse the wound by flushing it with 10-35 cc syringe with an 18-gauge angiocath to remove debris and bacteria using normal saline or dilute Betadine solution.
- Hand, puncture, and infected wounds or those more than 12 hours old may be closed by secondary intention.
- Use moisture-retentive dressings as indicated by the size and extent of wound left open. Dry dressings may be applied to injuries with closure by primary intention.
- Topical antibiotics may be indicated although systemic antibiotics are commonly prescribed for animal bites.
- Tetanus toxoid or immune globulin is routinely administered.

Spider Bites

Spider bites are frequently a misdiagnosis of a *Staphylococcus aureus* or MRSA infection, so unless the spider was observed, the wound should be cultured and antibiotics started. If the wound responds to the antibiotic, then it probably was not a spider bite. There are two main types of venomous spider bites:

- Producing neurological symptoms (Black widow)
- Producing local necrosis (brown recluse, yellow sac, and hobo spiders)

Treatment of spider bites universally includes first cleansing the wound and applying a cool compress. The body part should be elevated if possible.

Black widow bite treatment includes:

- Narcotic analgesics
- Nitroprusside to relieve hypertension
- Calcium gluconate 10% solution IV for abdominal cramps
- Latrodectus antivenin for those with severe reaction

Necrotic/ulcerated bites (brown recluse, etc.) treatment includes the following considerations:

- There is no consensus on the best treatment as ulceration caused by the venom may be extensive and surgical repair with grafts may be needed.
- Treatment as for other necrotic ulcers, with moisture retentive dressings as indicated.

Snake Bites

About 45,000 snake bites occur in the United States each year, about 8,000 of which are venomous. In the United States, about 25 species of snakes are venomous. There are 2 types of snakes that can cause serious injury, classified according to the type of fangs and venom.

Coral Snakes

Coral snakes have short fixed permanent fangs in the upper jaw and venom that is primarily neurotoxic, but may also have hemotoxic and cardiotoxic properties:

- Wounds show no fang marks but there may be scratches or semi-circular markings from teeth.
- There may be little local reaction, but neurological symptoms may range from mild to acute respiratory and cardiovascular failure.

Treatment includes:

- Cleanse the wound thoroughly of dirt and debris and leave it open or cover with dry dressing.
- Antibiotics are not usually needed.
- Administer antivenin immediately even without symptoms, which may be delayed.
- Administer tetanus toxoid or immune globulin.

PIT VIPERS

A second type of snake that can cause serious injury are pit vipers, including rattlesnakes, copperheads, and cottonmouths. These snakes have erectile fangs that fold until they are aroused, and their venom is primarily hemotoxic and cytotoxic but may have neurotoxic properties.

- Wounds usually show 1-2 fang marks.
- Edema may begin immediately or may be delayed up to 6 hours.
- Pain may be severe.
- There may be a wide range of symptoms, including hypotension and coagulopathy with defibrination that can lead to excessive blood loss, depending upon the type and amount of venom.
- There may be local infection and necrosis.

Treatment includes:

- Cleanse the wound thoroughly and apply dressings as indicated.
- Administer tetanus toxoid or immune globulin.
- Administer analgesics, such as morphine sulphate.
- Avoid NSAIDs and aspirin because of anticoagulation properties.
- Mark edema every 15 minutes.
- Administer antivenin therapy if indicated (observation for serum sickness if horse serum used).
- Administer prophylactic antibiotics for severe tissue necrosis.
- Administer platelets, plasma, or packed RBCs for coagulopathy.

ALLIGATOR BITES

Alligators are found in 10 coastal states in the southeastern United States with the largest population in Florida, where most injuries are reported. Animals between 4-8 feet often bite once and release, but larger animals may bite repeatedly, engaging in typical biting and feeding activities, and resulting in severe injury, amputations, or death. Most wounds involve the limbs, with the hands and arms the most frequently bitten. Treatment includes:

- Treatment for shock and blood loss.
- Apply pressure to the wound.
- Retrieve the amputated limbs if possible.
- Flush the wound with copious amounts of normal saline to reduce contamination.
- Collect wound cultures.
- Administer prophylactic broad-spectrum antibiotics for Gram negative organisms, such as *Aeromonas hydrophila* and *Clostridium.*
- Observe for signs of infection, such as erythema, cellulitis, exudate, necrosis.
- Administer tetanus toxoid or immune globulin.
- Repair fractures.
- Surgical repair and debridement as indicated with wounds usually healing by secondary intention or delayed primary closure.

Management of Mechanical Trauma

Mechanical trauma may result in stripping of the epidermis and sometimes the dermis of the skin or lacerations. Mechanical trauma may occur from tape removal or blunt trauma, such as colliding with furniture. Treatment includes:

- Recognize fragile skin and treat it carefully.
- Apply emollients, skin sealants, and skin barriers as indicated.
- Apply and remove tape appropriately.
- Avoid adhesives when possible.
- Use hydrocolloids, SteriStrips, and transparent dressings to stabilize flaps.

Management of Chemical Trauma

Chemical trauma may be caused by leakage or incontinence of body fluids, such as urine, feces, and exudate, or chemicals applied to the skin, such as lotions, iodine, soap, organic solvents, acids, and adhesives. Reactions to irritant contact dermatitis may vary widely, from an itching rash similar to allergic contact dermatitis to cracks and fissures in the skin, especially on the hands, or denudement of skin, often in the perineal area. The skin reaction may be rapid and extremely painful. Treatment includes:

- Identify the irritant and eliminate its contact with skin.
- Gently cleanse the skin to remove the irritant, avoiding further skin irritation.
- Use skin sealants or skin barriers as indicated to protect the skin and allow healing.
- Use appropriate skin care products and containment devices.
- Monitor dressings and peri-wound condition daily.

Wound Classification Systems

Classification of Wounds by Cause

Wounds can be classified in various ways. The most common classification of wounds is that according to cause:

- **Vascular wounds:** Vascular changes can result in wounds that occur most commonly in the lower extremities, such as those that result from arterial insufficiency and ischemia, those that relate to changes in the lymphatic system, and those related to venous insufficiency.
- **Neuropathic wounds:** Neuropathic changes that occur with chronic diseases, such as diabetes, and chronic alcoholism can decrease sensation and circulation, resulting in ulcerations.
- **Pressure injuries:** Shear friction and pressure, especially over bony prominences such as the sacral area and heels, causes erosion of the tissue.
- **Traumatic wounds:** Trauma often results in contaminated wounds.
- **Surgical wounds:** Surgery can result in wounds that are originally contaminated or originally clean, depending upon the type of surgery and the reason.
- **Infected wounds:** Inflammation and infection may result in deteriorating wounds or fistulas.
- **Self-inflicted wounds:** Vary widely, from minor cuts to traumatic gunshot wounds.
- **Dysfunctional healing wounds:** Hypergranulation/keloid formation can change the character of a wound and prevent adequate healing.

Staging System for Pressure Injuries

Pressure-related injuries result from pressure with or without shear and/or friction over bony prominences. The National Pressure Injury Advisory Panel developed a staging system to ensure that definitions for pressure injuries were standardized:

- **Suspected deep tissue injury**: Skin discolored, intact or blood blister
- **Stage I**: Intact skin with non-blanching reddened area
- **Stage II**: Abrasion or blistered area without slough but with partial-thickness skin loss
- **Stage III**: Deep tissue injury with exposed subcutaneous tissue; tunneling or undermining may be evident with or without slough or epibole (rolling inward of wound edge)
- **Stage IV**: Deep tissue injury, full thickness, with necrosis into muscle, bone, tendons, and/or joints
- **Unstageable**: Eschar and/or slough prevents staging prior to debridement

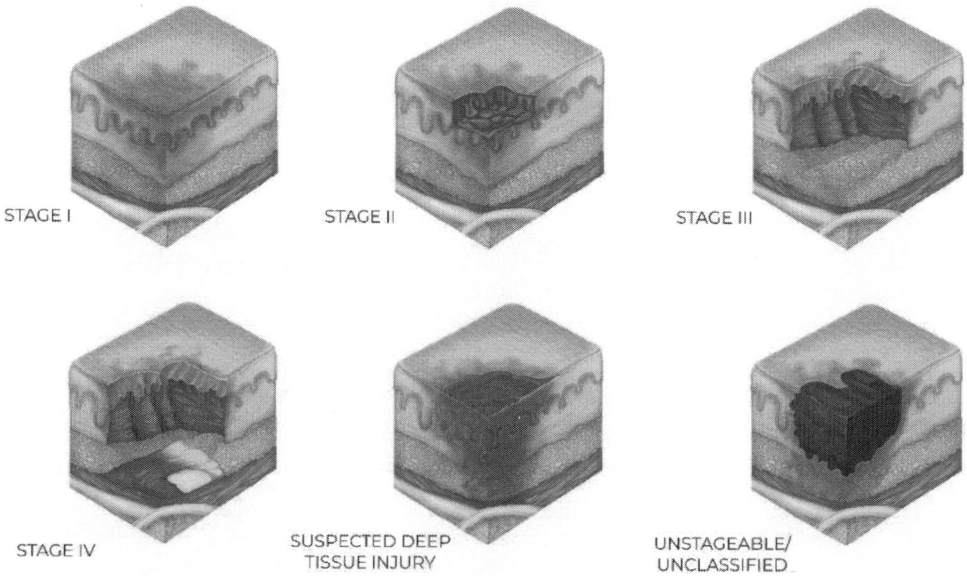

Modified Wagner Ulcer Classification System for Foot Ulcers

The modified Wagner Ulcer Classification System divides foot ulcers into six grades, based on lesion depth, osteomyelitis or gangrene, infection, ischemia, and neuropathy:

- **Grade 0**: At risk but no open ulcers
- **Grade 1**: Superficial ulcer, extending into subcutaneous tissue; superficial infection with or without cellulitis
- **Grade 2**: Full-thickness ulcer to tendon or joint with no abscess or osteomyelitis
- **Grade 3**: Full-thickness ulcer that may extend to bone with abscess, osteomyelitis, or sepsis of joint and may include deep plantar infections, abscesses, fasciitis, or infections of tendon sheath
- **Grade 4**: Gangrene in one area of foot, but the foot is salvageable
- **Grade 5**: Gangrene of entire foot, requiring amputation

While this classification system is useful in predicting outcomes, it does not contain information about the size of the ulcer or the type of infection, so it should be only one part of an assessment, as more detailed information is needed to fully evaluate an ulcer.

University of Texas Diabetic Foot Wound Classification System

The University of Texas created a wound classification system to account for the shortcomings of the Wagner classification system. Although the Wagner system is still used today, it has limitations at predicting outcome after grade 3 and lacks certain aspects of the wound assessment, making it less comprehensive in nature. The University of Texas wound classification system considers the wound's depth and infection status, as well as the presence of peripheral arterial occlusive disease, and evaluates the wound by both grade (0 through 3) and Stage (A, B, C, or D), which are defined as follows:

Stage	Grade 0	Grade 1	Grade 2	Grade 3
A	Lesion (pre- or post-ulcerative) is completely epithelialized	Ulcer is superficial and does not involve tendon or bone	Ulcer penetrates to the tendon	Ulcer penetrates to the bone/joint space
B	Infection present	Infection present	Infection present	Infection present
C	Ischemia present	Ischemia present	Ischemia present	Ischemia present
D	Both infection and ischemia present	Both infection and ischemia present	Both infection and ischemia present	Both infection and ischemia present

S(AD) SAD Classification System

S(AD) SAD stands for Size (Area and Depth), Sepsis, Arteriopathy, and Denervation. The S(AD) SAD classification system for lower-extremity neuropathic disease is one of many that builds upon the original or modified Wagner classification system and assigns a 0-3 grade based on 5 categories: area, depth, sepsis, arteriopathy, and denervation.

- **Grade 0**: No pathology is evident.
- **Grade 1**: Ulcer is <10 mm^2, involving subcutaneous tissue with superficial slough or exudate, diminution or absence of pulses, and reduced sensation.
- **Grade 2**: Ulcer is 10-30 mm^2, extending to tendon, joint, capsule, or periosteum with cellulitis, absence of pulses except for neuropathy dominant ulcers that have palpable pedal pulses.
- **Grade 3**: Ulcer is >30 mm^2, extending to bones and/or joints; seen with osteomyelitis, gangrene, and Charcot's foot.

This grading system is useful, but as with most other classification systems, it doesn't provide a simple way to distinguish those wounds that follow an atypical pattern or may be consistent with the grade in some areas and inconsistent in others.

CEAP Classification for Chronic Venous Disorders

Clinical (C0-C6)

- 0: No apparent venous disease
- 1: Telangiectasia/reticular veins
- 2: Varicose veins
- 3: Edema
- 4: Skin changes
- 5: Healed ulcer
- 6: Active ulcer

Etiologic

- E_C: Congenital
- E_P: Primary
- E_S: Secondary
- E_N: No cause identified

Anatomic distribution

- A_S: Superficial veins
- A_D: Deep veins
- A_P: Perforating veins
- A_N: No location identified

Pathophysiological classification

- P_R: Reflux
- P_O: Obstruction
- $P_{R,O}$: Reflux and obstruction
- P_N: No pathophysiology identified

Wound Infections

Stages of Wound Infection

The skin contains natural flora that cause no problem with intact skin, but if the skin barrier is breached, these microorganisms can migrate in to an open wound. Additionally, some pathogens, such as *Staphylococcus aureus,* are endemic to hospital environments and can contaminate wounds. Furthermore, **bioburden** (the presence of necrotic tissue and debris that prevent epithelialization from occurring) contributes to the development of infection in the wound.

There is a continuum to the **infectious process**:

- **Colonization** occurs when microorganisms replicate. There may be superficial signs of infection, but this phase is not pathogenic and should not be treated with antibiotics.
- **Critical colonization** occurs when the bioburden increases, arresting healing of the wound. Wounds may appear red and clean but lack granulation. The infection remains localized, and there is no systemic response. Topical antibiotics may be used at this phase.
- **Infection** occurs when the microorganisms invade the tissue and there is a systemic response. Acute wounds show signs of inflammation, but chronic wounds may only exhibit increased pain, exudate, or further delay in healing. Cultures and sensitivities should be done to ascertain the correct treatment.

Assessment of Wound Infection

There are a number of different aspects to the assessment for wound infection:

- **Patient history**: A complete history is critical. Any prior hospitalizations or recent surgeries should be noted as well as medication history. The history should show when and how the wound first occurred to help determine if the wound is acute or chronic. Co-morbidities should be noted as well as age and cognitive, functional, and nutritional status.
- **Examination**: A complete assessment of the wound, noting wound characteristics and drainage, should be done along with a careful and complete physical examination.
- **Laboratory testing**: Laboratory findings provide indications of the type and extent of infection and should include the complete blood count to determine if there is elevation of the white blood count. Wound cultures and sensitivities should be done to identify the microorganism and treatment. CT scans may be done to identify abscesses.

Review Video: Wound Infections
Visit mometrix.com/academy and enter code: 761736

Surgical Site Infections

CDC Criteria for Incisional and Organ/Space Surgical Site Infections

The CDC classifies surgical site infections as superficial incisional, deep incisional, or organ/space, depending on the severity of the infection:

- **Superficial incisional**:
  - Occurs within 30 days of surgery
  - Purulent discharge evident, organisms isolated, signs of infection and wound opened by surgeon, or diagnosis by physician
- **Deep incisional**:
  - Occurs within 30 days of surgery if no implant is in place, or 1 year if an implant is in place
  - Purulent discharge evident, signs of infections and incision dehisces or is deliberately opened by physician
  - Abscess or other evidence of infection found on examination, radiology, or histopathology
  - Diagnosis by physician
- **Organ/space**:
  - Occurs within 30 days of surgery if no implant is in place, or 1 year if an implant is in place if infection appears related
  - Infection involves any part of the body (organs, tissues) manipulated during surgery
  - Purulent discharge evident from drain to organ/space, organisms isolated from fluids or tissue in organ space, abscess in area, or diagnosis by physician

Risk Factors for Surgical Site Infections

Risk factors should be carefully assessed to determine the likelihood of surgical site infections:

- **Duration of surgery**: Surgeries more than 2 hours in length increase risk.
- **Co-morbidity**: Some conditions, such as diabetes mellitus or skin disease in surgical area, predispose patients to infection.
- **Steroids**: Immunosuppressive response allows infection.
- **Malnutrition**: Nutrients needed for healing are lacking.
- **Recent surgery**: Each procedure increases risk.
- **Extended hospitalization**: Risk increases with length of hospitalization prior to surgery.
- ***Staphylococcus aureus***: Nasal colonization or presence on skin allows bacteria to migrate to wound.
- **Remote infection**: Infection anywhere else in the body poses risk.
- **Prior radiation**: Radiation therapy compromises tissue and delays healing, allowing for infection to occur more easily.
- **Old/young**: The very young and elderly are more easily infected.
- **Circulatory impairment**: Hypoxemia or localized impairment, such as with peripheral vascular disease, compromise tissue. Smoking interferes with circulation as well.

Vital Signs Indicating Systemic Infection Leading to Sepsis

Infections caused by viruses, fungi, bacteria, and parasites can lead to sepsis, especially in the immunocompromised or those who have injuries that impair the body's defense, such as large contaminated wounds or burns. Signs of wound infection, such as warmth, pain, odorous exudate, and pus, or changes in condition should prompt one to check the patient's vital signs for typical **signs that may indicate sepsis**:

- Hyperthermia with temperature >38 °C OR hypothermia with temperature <35 °C
- Temperature changes possibly occurring with chills
- Increased respiratory rate (>20/min)
- Increased pulse rate
- Hypotension with falling blood pressure and <90 mmHg systolic or >40 mmHg decrease from normal reading

The symptoms indicating sepsis may relate to the underlying infection, such as pneumonia or meningitis, so symptoms may vary considerably, depending upon the causative agent and the site of infection. Some people may exhibit few symptoms while others may develop severe symptoms.

Risk Assessment

Determining Risk from Patient's Medical History

A thorough medical history will uncover information about diseases that have an impact on the condition of the skin:

- Medication and supplements taken, allergies, and hygiene practices should be noted as well as soaps, lotions, and other skin care products used.
- Environmental conditions and exposure to agents that are harmful to the skin at home, at work, or during recreation are important.
- Previous skin problems, problems with wound healing, and hereditary conditions affecting the skin should be determined.
- Nutritional status and dietary habits should be discussed.
- Symptoms of vascular problems should be noted.
- The patient's support system is important if help is needed for ADLs.
- Past exposure to radiation is noted along with the location, duration, strength of radiation, and effects on the skin.
- Financial status and health care insurance status of those who require wound care must also be considered.

Impact of Smoking on Peripheral Circulation

Smoking is a primary cause of lower extremity arterial disease, with diagnosis of disease 10 years before non-smokers. The effects of smoking on peripheral circulation include:

- Smoking decreases the blood flow to the extremities by causing arterial spasms that last 1 hour or longer.
- Carboxyhemoglobin from smoke is thought to harm the lining of the blood vessels, thus encouraging thrombus formation.
- Platelet function is also affected, increasing the formation of blood clots.
- Prostacyclin, a prostaglandin that inhibits platelet aggregation and causes vasodilation, is inhibited in production by smoking.

- Smoking increases the rate of atherosclerosis, decreases HDL, increases blood pressure, and decreases clotting time.
- The risk of claudication is nine times higher for smokers. Those with intermittent claudication who quit do not usually progress to having pain at rest.

Risk Factors for Pressure Injuries

Braden Scale for Pressure Injury Risk Assessment

The Braden scale is a risk assessment tool that has been validated clinically as predictive of the risk of patient's developing pressure injuries. It was developed in 1988 by Barbara Braden and Nancy Bergstrom and is in wide use. The scale scores 6 different areas with 1-4 points.

- **Sensory perception**
    - 1. Completely limited (unresponsive to pain or limited ability to feel)
    - 2. Very limited (responds to painful stimuli and moans)
    - 3. Slightly limited (responds to verbal commands but limited communication)
    - 4. No impairment
- **Moisture**
    - 1. Moist constantly
    - 2. Very moist (linen change each shift)
    - 3. Occasionally moist (linen change each day)
    - 4. Rarely moist
- **Activity**
    - 1. Bed bound
    - 2. Chair bound
    - 3. Walks occasionally (short distances)
    - 4. Walks frequently
- **Mobility**
    - 1. Completely immobile
    - 2. Very limited (makes occasional slight position changes)
    - 3. Slightly limited (makes frequently slight position changes)
    - 4. No limitations
- **Usual nutrition pattern**
    - 1. Very poor (eats < half of meals and has inadequate protein intake, and hydration)
    - 2. Inadequate (eats about half of food with 3 protein servings or not enough liquid or tube feeding)
    - 3. Adequate (eats more than half of meals and 4 protein servings)
    - 4. Excellent
- **Friction and shear** (3 parameters only)
    - 1. Problem moving (skin frequently slides down sheets, needs help to move)
    - 2. Potential problem (moves weakly or needs some assistance, skin slides somewhat during moves)
    - 3. No apparent problem

The scores for all six items are totaled, and a risk is assigned according to the number:

- 23 (best score) excellent prognosis, very minimal risk.
- ≤16 break point for risk of pressure injury (will vary somewhat for different populations).
- 6 (worst score) prognosis is very poor, strong likelihood of developing pressure injury.

Braden Q and Braden QD Scales

The Braden Q scale is the pediatric version of the Braden scale, meant to rate risk for pediatric patients. This scale uses all six subscales from the original Braden scale, and adds a seventh for **tissue perfusion/oxygenation** which is broken down as follows:

- 1. Extremely compromised (hypotensive or unable to tolerate repositioning)
- 2. Compromised (normal blood pressure with oxygen saturation <95% OR hemoglobin <10 mg/dL OR capillary refill >2 seconds with a serum pH of <7.4)
- 3. Adequate (normal blood pressure with oxygen saturation <95% OR hemoglobin <10 mg/dL OR capillary refill >2 seconds with a serum pH that is normal)
- 4. Excellent (normal blood pressure, oxygen saturation, hemoglobin, and capillary refill)

In 2018, the Braden Q scale was updated to the Braden QD scale. The Braden QD scale has 7 subscales, each rated from 0 to 2 (except for the *number of medical devices* subscale, which is a total count of all medical devices, with a max of 8). 0 indicates no problem, 1 indicates potential problem, and 2 indicates a problem. The 7 subscales are as follows:

- Mobility
- Sensory perception
- Friction and shear
- Nutrition
- Tissue perfusion and oxygenation
- Number of medical devices
- Repositionability/skin protection

A score of 13 or higher places the patient at risk for a pressure injury.

Norton Scale

Often compared to the Braden Scale, the Norton Scale is another scale measuring risk for pressure injuries in the adult population. This scale was created in 1962, before the Braden Scale, and has been criticized for being less predictive of pressure injuries than the Braden Scale. Five categories are rated, with scores stratifying risk as low (>18), medium (14-18), high (10-14), and very high (<10). Categories are as follows:

- Physical Condition
    - Good (4)
    - Fair (3)
    - Poor (2)
    - Very Bad (1)
- Mental Condition
    - Alert (4)
    - Apathetic (3)
    - Confused (2)
    - Stuporous (1)
- Activity
    - Ambulatory (4)
    - Walks with help (3)
    - Chairbound (2)
    - Bedfast (1)

- Mobility
    - Full (4)
    - Slightly impaired (3)
    - Very limited (2)
    - Immobile (1)
- Incontinence
    - None (4)
    - Occasional (3)
    - Usually urinary (2)
    - Urinary and fecal (1)

COMMON RISK FACTORS FOR PRESSURE INJURIES

The Centers for Medicare and Medicaid Services (CMS) established a list of common risk factors for pressure injuries. Many people present with more than one risk factor. Assessment should include evaluation of risks for following:

- Impairment or decreased mobility or functional ability that prevents a person from changing position.
- Co-morbid conditions affecting circulation or metabolism, such as renal disease, diabetes, and thyroid disease.
- Drugs that interfere with healing, such as corticosteroids.
- Impaired circulation, such as generalized atherosclerosis or arterial insufficiency of lower extremity, reducing tissue perfusion.
- Patient refusal of care, increasing risk (positioning, hygiene, nutrition, hydration, skin care).
- Cognitive impairment that prevents the patient from reporting discomfort or cooperating with care.
- Fecal and/or urinary contamination of skin, usually related to incontinence.
- Under nutrition or frank malnutrition and/or dehydration.
- Previous healed pressure injuries. Healed pressure injuries that were Stage III or IV may deteriorate and breakdown again.

IMMOBILITY

Immobility increases the chance of pressure injury development by reducing the voluntary shifting of pressure off of bony prominences. The patient who is unable to move independently must rely on others to change position. Reduced sensory perception of pain adds to the risk. The patient who has restricted mobility may not be able to maintain posture when upright, allowing the body to slump and increasing the chance of shearing as the body succumbs to gravity causing the skeleton to slide downwards as the skin of the sacrum remains in place due to friction against the bed. When caregivers reposition the patient without the aid of a lifting sheet friction against bed linens occurs and increases the chance of skin breakdown. Turning and repositioning plans must be developed for patients who are unable to change position voluntarily. Reconditioning exercises are needed for those who are debilitated but have intact muscular and sensory capabilities.

IMPAIRED COGNITION

The patient with impaired cognition is unable to translate sensory input that warns them of impending problems. They are not alert enough to shift position or signal the need for help from others to do so. They may not recognize sensations of pain, the location of the pain, or the connection between pain and the need to reposition. They do not associate the need for proper fluid and nutritional intake with their health status. They are dependent upon others for all activities of daily living and are often unable to recognize or stop harmful activity. They may engage in activities, such as picking or scratching the skin, without realizing that they are causing damage. They may be incontinent of stool and feces, and the added risk factor of moisture adds to the risk of skin breakdown.

Populations at Risk for Pressure Injuries

Populations at risk for pressure injuries include the following;

- The **elderly**, especially those with impairment of mobility or changes to the skin, experience the most pressure injuries, often associated with hospitalization or long-term care. For those admitted to long-term care facilities, 10-18% have at least one pressure injury on admission.
- People with **spinal cord injuries** are at risk because of loss of sensation. Studies have shown that approximately one-third of patients with spinal cord injuries will develop a pressure injury at some time.
- **Children** who are hospitalized are also at risk, but rates vary widely depending upon the child's condition and the setting. Rates may be as high as 27% in pediatric care units and as high as 20% in neonatal intensive care units. Pressure injuries usually occur within the first 2 days after admission.
- **Surgical patients** have pressure injury rates of 4-45%, depending on age, nutrition, and co-morbidities. Tissue damage may not be evident for up to 3 days after injury.

Risk Factors From Lower Extremity Wounds

A lower extremity wound can impact the person's ability to function physically, and put the patient at risk for additional wounds:

- Pain and discomfort may limit the amount of standing and ambulation.
- Enforced immobility, such as being on bed rest with leg elevated, severely constrains physical functioning, leading to pressure injuries.
- Bowel function may be compromised, and constipation from decreased activity is common. Antibiotic therapy associated with the wound may cause diarrhea, which leads to skin breakdown.
- The person's quality of sleep and energy level may be decreased, causing fatigue at home and at work.
- Side effects from antibiotics and other medications also may impair the ability to function.
- The ability to perform ADLS can also be affected by pain, limited mobility, bulky dressings, and fatigue or other symptoms and side effects.

The care provider should assess the patient for these problems and help to find solutions. The care provider should also assess this patient for new wounds. Many of these patients will need help with ADLs at home.

Risks Factors for Medical Adhesive-Related Skin Injury and Skin Tears

Medical adhesive-related skin injury (MARSI) occurs when the superficial layers of the skin are peeled away when adhesive is removed. Other evidence of MARSI may include skin tears, erythema, itching, and vesicular lesions. MARSI persists more than 30 minutes after the adhesive is removed and may result from traumatic injury to the tissue (such as epidermal stripping or tension injury), contact dermatitis, or allergic dermatitis. Risk factors include age (those of older age and neonates are at higher risk), and history of dermatologic disorders, malnutrition, dehydration, and underlying medical conditions.

Skin tears occur when layers of the skin are peeled away or separate from underlying tissue. Risk factors include older age, corticosteroid therapy, impaired mobility, and cognitive impairment. Skin tears are categorized with the **Payne-Martin Classification System**:

1. Skin tear (linear full thickness or flap partial thickness) leaves avulsed skin adequate to cover wound. Tears may be linear or flap-type.
2. Skin tear with loss of partial thickness, involving either scant (<25% of epidermal flap over tear is lost) to moderate-large (>25% of dermis in tear is lost).
3. Skin tear with complete loss of tissue, involving a partial-thickness wound with no epidermal flap.

Documenting on Wound Assessment

Patient Care Documentation

Patient documentation provides a legal record of patient status and care given. It acts as a communication tool between healthcare providers in their efforts to meet patient needs and ensure the best outcome. It serves as a record of services ordered and services given for billing purposes. Documentation also provides history of previous disease and treatments for reference. Allergies or sensitivities that may impact the patient's condition or treatments are recorded through documentation as well. Entries must always be precise, thorough, factual, and legible. Information must be updated as needed so that the record reflects the current status of the patient during the hospital stay. These principles also apply to care given in clinics, the doctor's office, or during a home health visit.

Documentation of Admission Skin Assessment

A pressure injury that develops after 24 hours in a facility is generally considered to be acquired at that facility. Therefore, it is crucial to conduct a thorough skin assessment documentation at the time of admission. The problem comes when an innocent looking bruise present on admission develops into a full-blown pressure injury. Therefore, one should utilize the new definition of deep tissue injury in the guidelines by the National Pressure Injury Advisory Panel (NPIAP) when assessing skin status on admission and designate any area with maroon or purple skin or a blood-filled blister as a suspected deep tissue injury on admission. This designation should also be given to any areas of skin that are painful to the patient, appear changed in texture and firmness from the surrounding skin, or are warmer and cooler. A good-quality photograph of these areas may be included, according to facility policy, with written documentation.

Ongoing Wound or Tissue Injury Documentation

The primary documentation of the wound or injury at the time of presentation for care must be as thorough as possible to establish the baseline to measure the success or failure of healing interventions. The size (length, width, depth), extent (tunneled, undermined), character (granulation, slough, eschar), color (red, pink, black), odor (none, slight, foul), and degree and type of drainage should be initially documented for baseline measurement and then regularly documented to show changes. Photographs should be taken. Consistent photography is valid documentation, but sporadic photography is not. Each photo must be dated and matched with a written description of the wound at the time of the photo. Documentation on wound progress should occur daily with a thorough assessment at least weekly. Documentation should be done in a consistent manner to indicate that care is consistent.

Tools to Monitor and Document Wound Healing

There are three tools used to help monitor wound healing. They all assess the wound, and two also assess the peri-wound areas. The tools all differ in the manner that they are set up. They allow the person doing the assessment to assign a numerical score to the wound:

- **The Sussman Wound Healing Tool (SWHT*)*** is used by physical therapists to measure the results of various PT treatments on pressure injuries. Changes in the wound are classified as "good" or "not good" for healing.
- **The Pressure Ulcer Scale for Healing (PUSH)** was developed by the National Pressure Injury Advisory Panel (NPIAP) and measures the surface area of the wound, the amount of exudate, and the wound appearance.
- **Bates-Jensen Wound Assessment Tool (BWAT)**, formerly known as Pressure Sore Status Tool (PSST), assesses 13 wound characteristics and grades them from best to worst.

Documentation of Wound Care Process

Documentation of the wound care process should include the following elements:

- **Medication Administration**: Document the name of the medication, the dosage and the route of administration, site of administration (such as for IM injections) as well as the time of administration and follow-up response (such as relief of pain after analgesia) and times of monitoring.
- **Wound Progression (Healing)**: The description must be accurate, including the location, size, depth, stage, and character of the wound, supplemented with photographs (especially at the beginning of treatment and after debridement) or drawings. Changes should be noted at each dressing change and physician visit or intervention, such as debridement. Any complicating factors, such as PAD, and interventions to alleviate them should be documented. The plan of care with expected outcomes should be included.
- **Billing**: Documentation requirements must be met, including the reason for treatment. Documentation must support the service that is billed, and the correct ICD and CPT codes must be utilized for the institution.

Using Photographs to Document Wound Changes

Documenting wound changes with photographs is an issue of risk management, so facility-wide procedures must be in place regarding the use of photographs. Guidelines must specify:

- The type of camera and film that can be used. Some facilities mandate only Polaroid pictures because digital images can be manipulated. Others use digital cameras because of ease of entering pictures into computerized systems.
- Specific guidelines as to distance requirements indicating how many inches the camera should be from the wound
- Guidelines for including the date in the photograph and using measures (such as disposable rulers)
- Designation of staff allowed to photograph and training required
- Types of wounds/conditions that may be photographed
- Consent form

A wound photo may be taken by any type of camera. Low-cost instant cameras may not deliver the close-up, clear, true color photo that is desired. Moderately priced digital cameras with as high a resolution as possible deliver the best quality photo and provide instant feedback.

Tips for Taking Photos of Wounds

Tips for taking photos of wounds:

- The correct distance from the wound should be verified using a measuring device, such as a length of string attached to the front of the camera (changed between patients).
- Lighting will affect the colors of the wound. A flash camera will give a blue color and incandescent light will give a yellow cast to the photo. Good ambient light is helpful.
- The patient should be positioned so only the wound is shown in the photo. Other parts of the body should be screened off with drapes. The patient's face should not be shown unless the wound is on the face.
- A ruler should be placed next to the wound to indicate wound size.
- A sign with patient identification and the date may be included in the photo.
- The patient position at the time of the photo should be documented for future reference.
- A written description of the wound must be included in the record with the photograph.

Photographic Wound Assessment Tool

The **Photographic Wound Assessment Tool (PWAT)** is a modification of the Bates-Jenson Wound Assessment Tool (BWAT). The tool contains 6 domains (areas) of information that can be determined from the photo:

- Edges of the wound
- Type of necrotic tissue
- Amount/degree of necrotic tissue
- Periwound color
- Evidence of granulation
- Evidence of epithelialization

Each domain is scored from 0 to 4, with a total resulting score that can range from 0 (healed) to 24. Serial photographs are taken on a regular schedule. Studies have shown that this photographic method of assessment is as accurate as bedside assessment of the wound, especially for pressure wounds as the BWAT is designed for pressure wounds rather than other types. PWAT provides a tool for telemedicine use when a clinician cannot be at the patient's bedside to evaluate a wound.

Intervention and Treatment

Pressure Redistribution

Tissue Interface Pressures

Tissue interface pressure is the amount of pressure exerted on the body by a surface that the body is lying or sitting on. Small sensors are placed between the patient and the surface to measure pressures in localized areas. The measurement is important to assess whether the pressure is great enough to occlude the capillaries in the area, increasing the risk of tissue ischemia and injury formation. The force that closes capillaries is 12-32 mmHg. This range is used as a comparison along with patient condition, skin condition, nutrition, and other factors to decide whether a support surface relieves enough pressure in a specific location on that particular patient. However, research has not demonstrated that there is a specific threshold at which pressure will cause harm, so the tissue interface pressure should only be used as a guide and not a substitute for observation.

Pressure Injury Prevention

Every patient should be assessed for **risk factors** for pressure injuries. These include immobility, inactivity, moisture and incontinence, poor nutritional state and intake, friction and shear, decreased sensation, mental status changes, fragile skin condition, and certain medications. Tools are available for assessing patient risk for pressure injuries, including the Gosnell Scale and the Braden Scale. Use of these scales provides consistency in assessment from patient to patient and can be used to assess changes in risk level as a result of interventions. Once the risk factors are defined, prevention can concentrate on alleviating these factors. Interventions are designed, and patient and family teaching is performed. Interventions are specific for each patient, disease status, and individual situation. Several solutions for risk factors are possible, and solutions must be individualized for the patient.

Turning and Repositioning to Reduce Pressure

Measures to reduce pressure include turning and repositioning.

- Goals for repositioning and a turning schedule of at least every 2 hours should be established for each individual, with documentation required.
- Devices, such as pillows or foam, should be used to correctly position patients so that bony prominences are protected and not in direct contact with each other.
- Re-position patients carefully to avoid friction or shear.
- Assistive devices should be used if necessary to move patients.
- Use chairs of correct size and height and use pressure relieving devices for the seats.
- Limit chair time for those who are acutely ill to no more than 2 hours.
- Patients should be taught or reminded to redistribute weight every 15 minutes. A timer may be used to remind patients.
- Use the 30° lateral position rather than the 90° side-lying position.

Positioning Strategies in the Bed and Chair

Passive repositioning should be performed on the patient in both the bed and the chair:

- **Bed**: When positioned on his or her side, the patient should be turned to a 30° laterally-inclined position rather than a 90° side-lying position, which puts pressure on the trochanter. Two people should use a turn sheet, draw sheet, and pillows to pull up in bed, turn, and position the patient. Pillows should be placed under the head, under the legs to keep heels off the bed, behind the back, and between the ankles and knees.
- **Chair**: Patients in chairs need repositioning hourly as well. The patient should be assisted to stand and sit down again. Small changes in seated patients include changing leg position from dependent to elevated. The body should be in proper alignment, using pillows or cushions if needed. Patients who are cognizant and able to shift position should be instructed to do so every 15 minutes while seated.

Use of Support Surfaces to Prevent Pressure Injuries

A support surface redistributes pressure to prevent pressure injuries and reduce shear and friction. There are various types of support surfaces for beds, examining tables, operating tables, and chairs. General use guidelines include:

- Pressure redistribution support surfaces should be used in beds, operating tables, and examining tables for at-risk individuals.
- Patients with multiple injuries or with stage II to stage IV injuries require support surfaces.
- Chairs should have gel or air support surfaces to redistribute pressure for chair bound patients, critically ill patients, and those who cannot move independently.
- Support surface material should provide at least an inch of support under areas to be protected when in use to prevent bottoming out. (Check by placing hand palm-up under overlay below the pressure point.)
- Static support surfaces are appropriate for patients who can change position without increasing pressure to an injury.
- Dynamic support surfaces are needed for those who need assistance to move or when static pressure devices provide less than an inch of support.

Categories of Support Surfaces

There are five elements that are used to categorize support surfaces:

- **Pressure redistribution** may be preventive (≤32 mmHg, but not consistently) or therapeutic (≤32 mmHg, consistently). Preventive devices are used for those at risk or with stage I or II injuries. Therapeutic devices are used for those with stage III and IV pressure injuries.
- **Device forms** are varied and may supplement or replace existing equipment. Devices include chair cushions, mattress overlays, pressure-reducing mattresses, and specialty bed systems used in place of traditional hospital beds.
- **Active support surfaces** are powered, requiring attachment to an electrical motor for utilization, (dynamic) or non-powered (static).
- **Medium** may be different types of foam, water, gels, or air.
- **Medicare reimbursement group**:
  - Group 1: Used as a preventive measure and includes overlays and mattresses.
  - Group 2: Used as a therapeutic measure and includes non-powered and powered overlays and mattresses.
  - Group 3: Used as a therapeutic measure and includes air-fluidized beds.

Functions of Support Surfaces

Support surfaces are designed for a number of functions:

- **Pressure redistribution** occurs through *immersion* (spreading the pressure out) and *envelopment* (conforming to shape without increasing pressure). The aim is to reduce pressure on the skin to less than the capillary closing pressure (<32 mmHg), but lower pressures may be necessary for elderly patients. *Interface pressure measurement* is measurement of the pressure exerted between the body and the support surface. This measurement is currently used to evaluate the pressure redistribution efficiency of devices although it has not been demonstrated through research that this measurement can predict clinical performance. Thin, flexible sensors are placed under the support surface and the patient and computerized readings indicate if the support surface is adequate. A number of new measurement devices are now marketed that show colored-coded computerized pictures demonstrating different levels of pressure.
- **Temperature control** is important because temperature increases can lead to skin breakdown. Skin temperature relates to the specific heat of the material in the support surface. Specific heat (the ability to conduct heat) varies considerably from one type of material to another. Air has a low specific heat, and water has a high specific heat. Material with high specific heat may conduct heat away from the body, decreasing skin temperature.
- **Moisture control** prevents moisture damage to skin, but there are wide ranges of materials in use in support surfaces. Some materials, such as rubber or plastic, may increase perspiration and moisture, while some porous materials, such as some foams, may reduce perspiration.
- **Friction/shear control** is more difficult to achieve although some surface coverings, such as those with Gortex, are purposely slick to decrease friction. However, proper positioning, lifting, and repositioning still must be done.

Redistribution Media

Water

Water in overlays or mattresses is a common redistribution medium. The water may flow between cells or may be in one large space. Weight floating on water is evenly distributed, so waterbeds provide good weight distribution, and they have good immersion qualities, so the patient's body sinks into the surface, which then molds to their body shape. While these devices are popular in the home, there are a number of disadvantages to their use in healthcare facilities:

- They require electricity and a heater to keep the correct temperature.
- Water is very heavy, so they are difficult to move and maneuver.
- Draining and filling is messy and time-consuming.
- They may leak if punctured or around connections.
- Water is pulled by gravity, so if the head of the bed is elevated, the water flows downward, leaving uneven distribution.
- Moving or repositioning patients on a water support surface can be difficult because of the constant movement of the water.

FOAM

Foam varies considerably according to density and indentation load definition (ILD). Foam can be closed-cell (resistant) or open cell (viscoelastic). The number of chemicals used in the manufacturing of polyurethane foam determines the weight and viscoelasticity. Higher densities have higher viscoelastic (molding) properties. Open-cell foam is temperature-sensitive, helping it to mold to the body as it reaches the patient's body temperature. The density number of foam indicates the weight per cubic foot. Firmness is determined by the ILD, which is the number of pounds of pressure needed to indent a 4-inch foam 25% of its thickness using an indentation of 50 square inches. (Body weight and pounds of pressure should not be confused.) Foam is relatively inexpensive and was one of the first support surfaces used. Overlays should be 3-4 inches thick with densities of 1.3-1.6, and ILD of about 30.

Foam also has some **disadvantages**:

- Increases skin temperature
- Has a short lifespan
- Loses fire-retardance if it gets wet

AIR

Non-powered (static) air redistribution devices are manufactured in various forms: cushions, pads, overlays, and mattresses. The **air-filled overlays** may have a single bladder or the multi-cells/cylinders, with multi-cell forms providing the most pressure redistribution. Most forms are reusable and are filled with pumps to levels prescribed by the manufacturer according to the size and weight of the individual. The air moves with the individual, and the degree of immersion determines the effectives of the device.

Powered (dynamic) alternating pressure overlays have cells or cylinders that are alternately inflated and deflated at prescribed intervals by way of a pump that is attached to the overlay. Air overlays must be checked frequently to ensure that there is adequate air filling. Disadvantages include susceptibility to shear when the bed is elevated and bottoming out. Air overlays are recommended only for those <250 pounds. The degree of temperature and moisture control depends on the covering.

Air-fluidized (high air loss) beds are special bed systems that have a high flow of air through silicon beads, originally designed for treatment of burn patients. As the air flows through the beads, it fluidizes them so that they move and provide support and redistribution of pressure in much the way water does. The beads are contained in a bathtub-like frame. The lower part of the body becomes immersed in the beads so that the person appears to be floating as the beads move about because of the air. The air-fluidized bed is most commonly used for patients with multiple pressure injuries, making positioning to avoid pressure on sores very difficult, or who have had surgery for myocutaneous flaps. These expensive beds provide a warm alkaline environment and a bactericidal effect. There is some indication that capillary perfusion may become occluded, resulting in pressure injuries, although existing injuries heal faster.

Low air loss beds, overlays, and cushions have porous surfaces that allow air that is pumped in the support surface to leak, so there is a continuous flow of air through the air pillows in the device. The air pressure in the pillows in the devices can be adjusted according to the individual needs. The low air loss bed systems provide better immersion than air overlays and the patient cannot bottom out if the device is properly maintained. The covers for the devices are usually made of nylon or polytetrafluoroethylene fabric, both of which minimize friction. Only linen coverings or special pads that are air-permeable should be used with low air loss devices so that the air can flow beneath the skin. Disadvantages are that the equipment is expensive and contraindicated for those with an unstable spine. The airflow in beds must be maintained properly or there is a danger of entrapment in the bed. Hypothermia sometimes occurs.

Gels

Gels, which consist of silicone elastomer, silicone, or polyvinyl chloride, are fluid emulsions used in the manufacture of numerous devices, such as chair cushions and other types of flotation pads, such as overlays for beds, operating tables, and exam tables. There are also gel mattress replacements. Gel flotation pads usually have covers that can be disinfected so they can be used by multiple patients, a factor in their versatility. They are relatively inexpensive and require no electricity. Gels provide protection against shear and have good immersion properties, molding well to the body shape and providing good pressure redistribution. There are, however, some **disadvantages**:

- They are heavy.
- The gel filling may break up over time, leading to uneven distribution.
- They are difficult to repair.
- They may increase body temperature.
- They are not suitable for moisture control.

Off-Loading

Off-loading is relief of pressure on an ulcerated area of the foot while walking. Meticulous effective wound care plus off-loading promotes rapid healing of foot ulcers or other pressure injuries. Any material used must be able to be compressed to half of its thickness to be effective. Pressure testing of the standing foot or insoles that conform to the patient's foot is used to identify areas needing off-loading. Temperature testing reveals areas with increased temperature indicating tissue trauma:

- Specialized inserts may be used inside a shoe, tailored to relieve pressure in areas as needed.
- Special shoes are designed for some patients to relieve pressure.
- Crepe soles may provide relief.
- The heel of a shoe may be modified to compensate for limited toe motion, a varus deformity, or a decreased arch.
- A wide shoe that allows 0.5-0.75 in above the toes is needed for neuropathic feet.
- Cast shoes, wedged shoes, healing sandals, and half shoes are all alternative shoes that may provide the proper off-loading for the patient's needs.

Total Contact Casts

Total contact casts (TCCs) are the most successful way to off-load a foot ulcer/pressure injury to promote healing. A TCC is like a fracture cast but differs in that more padding is used and the toes are covered. The cast is applied by a skilled person and molded closely to the foot and leg below the knee. This prevents any movement of the foot or leg within the cast. An ambulation platform is added to the cast to force the patient to off-load the injury while walking. The cast is confining, hot, and must be kept dry during bathing. It is very effective in healing wounds when combined with good wound care. It is changed every 1-2 weeks or more often for wound care or when edema is present.

Indications and Contraindications

Total contact casts (TCCs) are indicated for uninfected, debrided ulcers on the bottom of the foot when associated with neuropathy. TCC also is used to treat Charcot neuroarthropathy by reducing the stress of weight bearing.

TCC must not be used if infection or arterial insufficiency is present. Wounds with necrotic material can hide an abscess or osteomyelitis, so ulcers must undergo total debriding prior to TCC application. Open exposure of tendons, bones, or joint capsules is a contraindication to the use of a TCC. The skin must be free of active problems, and the patient must be free of allergies to cast materials. A TCC is contraindicated for obese patients or those who can't tolerate total enclosure of the foot and lower leg. It should not be used for those who are blind or who have an unsteady gait.

Removable Cast Walker to Off-Load a Foot Ulcer/Pressure Injury

A removable cast walker is a good alternative to a total contact cast (TCC) for the patient who can't tolerate the TCC or when it is contraindicated. It is easy to apply and removable for hygiene and more frequent wound care. It can be used to control edema in combination with compression therapy. There are several available for use that can be modified for the patient's particular needs. They are often made of plastic with foam inserts and padding and are secured with Velcro straps. Patient compliance is important when a removable cast-walking boot is used. An expensive custom-built ankle foot orthotic is sometimes used for difficult foot pathology. It consists of a molded polypropylene shell and acts as a splint. Another method is to mold a TCC and then cut a hinged opening to make it removable. It is then customized to off-load pressure. A cast shoe is placed over this splint for ambulation.

Walking Aides Used by Patients with Foot Ulcers

Patients with an unsteady gait and the elderly may need to have a walking aid when they use special shoes, a TCC and cast shoe, or an orthotic splint to heal an ulcer. Walking aides should be chosen with individual needs in mind. They must be customized to the person's height:

- A conventional walker with or without wheels may suffice.
- A 2-, 3-, or 4-wheeled walker with brakes may be more useful. They are available for use by both hands or just one hand. Some have seats so people can rest, but people must be cautioned to keep the walker braked when they are sitting.
- Quad canes are safer to use than a single-leg cane.
- Crutches may be suitable for younger patients with good upper body strength, but they must be fitted properly.

Considerations When Patient Needs Wheelchair Due to Foot Ulcers

The patient who needs to be totally non-weight bearing may need a wheelchair to allow mobility instead of being confined to bed with the attendant problems caused by immobility. The chair should be fitted by measuring the patient's seat depth, seat width, seat-to-foot support height, seat to top of sacrum for lumbar support, and height of backrest. The height of armrests must also be determined. Seat back height may need to be increased to accommodate special seat padding to reduce pressure on the ischial tuberosities. The leg rests may need to be elevated so they must be of the proper height and length and padded. The patient may need upper body strength training and must have training for proper wheelchair mobility and safe transfers into and out of the wheelchair.

Wound Preparation

Closure of Dead Space

Dead space is the defect of soft tissue left behind after debridement or excision of a space-occupying lesion. Dead space may also occur if portions of the wound separate beneath the skin after primary closure, leaving an open pocket if air/fluid becomes trapped between tissue layers. Closure of the dead space is essential because it promotes healing and decreases the risk of infection. Treatment options vary depending on the location, extent of the dead space, and the cause, but may include application of a compression bandage (using care not to apply excessive pressure that may impair oxygenation), insertion of a drain (open or closed, active or passive), and/or aspiration of fluid contents (seroma) of the dead space. Negative pressure wound therapy may be utilized for large wounds. Dead spaces open to the surface should be completely filled with suitable wound packing material (depending on the extent of drainage) but should be lightly packed so as to avoid pressure on healthy tissue. Patients may need to restrict activity during treatment for dead space.

Wound Edge Optimization

Chronic wounds may take weeks or months to heal, so wound edge optimization is essential to healing. If the wound edges are not advancing or there are indications of undermining or deterioration, this may indicate that the wound cells are nonresponsive and that there are abnormalities of protease activities. Wound optimization methods include careful wound assessment and adequate debridement of the wound to remove necrotic tissue through sharp excision or enzymatic debridement, such as with collagenase, which debrides and promotes epithelialization. Maintaining appropriate moisture balance is also important as excessive moisture may cause maceration and deterioration of the wound, while inadequate moisture may result in desiccation of the wound and slowed epithelialization. The choice of dressing, therefore, may affect the healing process. If infection occurs appropriate antimicrobials (systemic or topical) may be necessary. In some cases, bioengineered skin or skin grafts may be appropriate. Additionally, edema slows healing, increases the risk of bacterial colonization, and must be controlled, such as through compression therapy. Wound exudate should be controlled because exudate, especially with chronic wounds, depresses cell proliferation (fibroblasts, keratinocytes).

Maintaining a Warm and Moist Wound Environment

One of the basic principles of current wound care is the use of occlusive dressings that keep the wound warm and moist. There are a number of reasons for keeping a healing wound warm and moist:

- **Reduction in dehydration** allows cells such as neutrophils and fibroblasts to carry out their functions in wound repair, as they require a moist environment. This also results in less cell death.
- **Angiogenesis** requires a moist environment and low oxygen tension, which is found in occlusive dressings.
- **Autolytic debridement** with proteolytic enzymes is enhanced in a moist environment.
- **Re-epithelization** of tissue occurs because the epidermal cells are able to spread across the surface of the wound.
- **Reduction in microorganisms, facilitated by the seal provided by occlusive dressings, decreases infection.**
- **Pain reduction** results from the protection of the nerve endings and the need for fewer dressing changes.

Periwound Skin Protection

The area extending about 4 cm from the wound edges is the periwound tissue, and it is especially vulnerable to irritation from drainage and adhesive. The periwound tissue should be evaluated for increased warmth and erythema as well as signs of maceration from exposure to exudate. Moisture-associated and adhesive associated skin damage can be prevented and treated by gentle cleansing of the periwound tissue with NS or water and application of a skin barrier. Moisture-retentive dressings help to keep the wound surface moist while avoiding excessive wetness and can wick fluid away from the periwound tissue. Dressing changes should be minimized to prevent stripping of periwound skin. Barriers may include:

- **Alcohol-based skin sealants**: Provide a sticky surface to help adhesives adhere and provide some skin protection. Available in wipes and spray.
- **Creams/Ointments**: May contain petrolatum, zinc oxide, or dimethicone and are applied in a thin layer to the skin and covered with absorptive dressings or applied in the perineal area to prevent skin irritation from incontinence.
- **Topical corticosteroids**: Used for allergic reactions, such as to adhesives.

Wound Cleansing

Wound Cleansing with Each Dressing Change

Microorganisms, contaminants, and cellular debris in a wound can significantly delay healing and increase inflammation. Antiseptics such as hydrogen peroxide, acetic acid, povidone-iodine, or sodium hypochlorite (Dakin solution) are toxic to developing fibroblasts and interfere with healing over time. They are sometimes used and rinsed with saline for a short period of time to control heavily infected wounds. The current standard is to use irrigation to deliver normal saline in a manner forceful enough to break the adhesion of debris to the wound bed yet gentle enough to prevent injury to developing cells. Pressures of at least 5-15 psi delivered by mechanical irrigators are needed for effective cleansing. Higher pressures can cause penetration of the fluid into tissues. Irrigation using a 12 mL syringe and a 22 G needle will deliver a force of 13 psi. The use of a 35 mL syringe and a 19 G needle will deliver 8 psi and is more effective than using a bulb syringe when mechanical irrigation is not available.

Cleansing a Wound by Soaking

Soaking is a beneficial way to cleanse a wound that has a large amount of necrotic debris or contamination. Contamination must be removed from new wounds to avoid excess inflammation that will delay wound healing. Soaking softens any necrotic tissue and helps to ease it away from the healthy tissue at the bottom of the wound bed. It also helps to loosen contaminants that are embedded in the wound. Antiseptic agents should not be used in the soaking solution. Soaking may be accomplished using any container that will hold the wound area, or by whirlpool. The container must be disinfected well prior to and after the soaking. It may take several soaks to remove tough, dry eschar, and once the necrotic material has been removed, soaking should be discontinued, as it will then delay healing.

Irrigating a Wound for Cleansing Purposes

When **irrigating a wound** for cleansing purposes, the area beneath the wound should be covered to prevent contamination of the bed linens:

1. Place a basin beneath the wound to catch the returned solution.
2. Wash hands and wear gloves.
3. Use pulsatile lavage or a syringe to deliver water or saline with a force of 5-15 psi to the wound bed. Using pressure >15 psi forcefully injects irrigating fluid into newly formed tissues and risks inoculating microorganisms into deeper tissues. Highly contaminated or infected wounds may require pressure at the higher range of 15 psi to cleanse. Use low pressure (5-8 psi) to cleanse healthy wounds so new capillaries are not damaged.
4. Flush undermined, tunneled areas well, and then massage over the area of tunneling or undermining to dislodge debris and encourage the fluid to return.
5. Repeat as needed until the return fluid is free of debris.
6. Finish by packing these areas as ordered.

Cleansing a Shallow Wound by Scrubbing

Scrubbing is sometimes combined with a cleansing solution to initially cleanse a wound to remove debris. It is best performed using a very porous, soft sponge and a nonionic surfactant cleansing solution to avoid damaging the wound bed as much as possible. Even so, damage to the wound bed is often unavoidable, so scrubbing may be done initially to a traumatic wound, but the practice should not be continued after the wound is clean and beginning to heal because it can disrupt the development of granulation tissue and damage areas of epithelialization. When scrubbing, one should begin cleansing in the center of the wound and work in a circle toward the edges of the wound, avoiding recleansing an area to prevent recontamination of the center of the wound.

Pulsed Lavage

Pulsed lavage (pulsatile high-pressure lavage) is irrigation of an infected or necrotic wound under pressure, using an electrically powered device. Normal saline is commonly used for lavage treatments, with the amount varying according to the size and amount of exudate on the wound. It is recommended that the pressure be 8-15 psi. The pressure can be varied as needed. While there is concern that higher pressure may inoculate tissue with bacteria, studies have not indicated this. Exposed blood vessels, graft sites, and muscle tissue should be avoided with the lavage treatments, and treatments should be discontinued if bleeding occurs with patients taking anticoagulants. Treatment is usually done 1-2 times daily. Both the hose and irrigating nozzle are intended for one-time use, so treatments can be expensive.

Wounds Requiring Pulsed Lavage

Pulsatile lavage can be used on almost any type of wound but is particularly indicated for the following:

- Clean wounds to encourage granulation and healing
- Wounds with delayed healing to encourage granulation and stimulate epithelialization
- Severely contaminated or infected wounds to reduce microorganisms in the wound bed
- Pre-graft wound preparation to remove any contamination, foreign material, or necrosis and provide an optimal graft surface
- Diabetic neuropathic ulcers to treat without damaging callus or fragile areas
- Sacral wounds to allow easy access and comfort (as opposed to sitting in whirlpool)
- Wounds with undermining and tunneling to effectively irrigate (using smaller, flexible irrigation wands)

Patients who have cardiac monitoring, urinary catheters, IV lines, or other invasive monitoring avoid compromise to these areas when they have bedside irrigation of wounds. Febrile patients do not experience core warming as they do in whirlpools.

Precautions

Aerosolization of microorganisms is possible during the use of pulsatile lavage with suction to cleanse wounds. The patient should wear a facemask, and all areas of the body, except for the wound, should be covered. The cleansing should be done in a ventilated private room with cupboards, drawers, and doors closed with no one else present. Waterproof mattresses or pads without surface tears should be used. Unnecessary equipment in the room should be stowed during irrigation since all exposed areas of the room must be disinfected after irrigation is done. Wheelchairs or transport stretchers should be removed from the room. The person performing pulsatile lavage should have full personal protective gear on, including hair and shoe coverings, face shields, mask, gown, and gloves. Suctioned fluids should be emptied into a toilet or designated commode. Disposable equipment should be disposed of as hazardous waste. Suction canisters should be disposable or sterilized after use if made of glass. Bed linens and towels used during lavage should be double bagged and laundered.

Hydrotherapy

Hydrotherapy, often in the form of whirlpool treatments to a limb or the whole body, is used to cleanse and debride wounds that are large with significant necrosis. Hydrotherapy is frequently used to treat burn injuries. Water is used at a temperature of 37 °C. Antiseptics are sometimes added to the water but can interfere with healing. Hydrotherapy has been implicated in a number of outbreaks of wound infections caused by cross-contamination; so many facilities have discontinued the use of whirlpools. Additionally, they are contraindicated for venous ulcers because vasodilation can increase edema. Diabetic patients may be insensitive to temperature, so therapy must be used cautiously. Wounds related to arterial insufficiency may not benefit. Whirlpool treatments do not appear to reduce surface bacteria of wounds, but rinsing the tissue after the treatment does. Equipment must be thoroughly disinfected between patients to prevent spread of infection.

Patient Safety Measures During Whirlpool Treatments

Whirlpools are used to cleanse wounds with a large amount of contamination or necrotic tissue. Small whirlpools are best for extremity wounds so the entire body does not need to be immersed. Water used in whirlpools should first be tested for the presence of microorganisms. If antiseptics are used in the water, the patient should wear a mask to avoid allergic reactions to aerosolized antiseptic or pneumonia from water vapor droplets. Additional **patient safety measures** include:

- Transfer the patient into and out of the whirlpool cautiously if a large whirlpool is used.
- Monitor vital signs before, during, and after whirlpool treatments and observe for fainting, dizziness, or altered mental status.
- Position the patient away from the jets to avoid damage to the wound or other tissues from the high pressure.
- Adjust or discontinue agitation if tissues are fragile.
- Rinse all body surfaces and the wound after whirlpool to remove antiseptics, contamination, and cellular debris. This is best done by a vigorous warm water rinsing or by showering.

Periwound Cleansing

The stratum corneum of the **periwound skin** is not as stable as normal skin. Periwound skin has more skin debris, such as water-insoluble proteins, amino acids, urea, ammonia, microorganisms, and cholesterol, than other tissue. Microorganisms up to 10 cm away from the wound edge can be more numerous and differ from those found in the wound bed, so cleansing prevents wound contamination. The microorganism level increases when the amount of protein on the periwound surface is increased. This area must be cleansed along with the wound when dressing changes are done. Cleansing reduces bacterial counts within and around the wound for about 24 hours. Normal saline may not remove these substances adequately. A skin cleanser that is mild and will not harm skin or strip away intercellular lipids may be used on the periwound area.

Compression Therapy

Indications for Compression Therapy

When edema is present, wounds are unable to receive adequate nutrients, immune defenses are decreased, and epithelialization is poor or nonexistent. Compression therapy is used to control edema when there are lymphatic or venous insufficiencies. Compression must be used consistently to improve these conditions. It increases venous return by compressing superficial venous capillaries and forcing the blood into deeper veins for transport back to the heart. This minimizes venous hypertension and superficial capillary leakage. Arterial studies must be performed prior to compression therapy to ensure an adequate arterial blood supply. Pulses are assessed and Doppler studies are performed if pulses are weak. The Doppler ankle arterial pressure is divided by the Doppler brachial arterial pressure to determine the Ankle/Brachial Index to assess peripheral arterial disease. Baseline measurements are done prior to beginning therapy to establish the circumference of the extremity at several points. Serial measurements then demonstrate the effectiveness of the compression therapy. Ambulation and exercise are combined with compression to maximize the removal of edema.

Static Compression Therapy

Static compression therapy is applying external graduated pressure to a lower extremity, from the ankle to the knee, to support the calf muscle and increase venous flow. Compression therapy is not curative, but is used as a preventive and therapeutic treatment to eliminate edema. It is contraindicated in those with heart failure or peripheral arterial disease as it may further impair compromised arterial circulation. Compression should not be used if the ankle brachial index (ABI) is <0.5. There are many different types of static compression products, and they should be chosen according to individual needs. They are graded according to the level of compression:

- **High level** provides therapeutic compression at 30-40 mmHg at the ankle. Some may provide pressure at 40-50 mmHg. ABI should be >0.8.
- **Low level** provides modified pressure up to 23 mmHg at the ankle. ABI must be >0.5 to <0.8. While this level is less than therapeutic, some authorities believe that even low levels of pressure provide some therapeutic benefit.

Elastic

There are many products and different types of elastic static compression therapy:

- **Layered wraps** (Profore, ProGuide, and Dynapress) combine both elastic and non-elastic layers in 2-4 layers with the inner layers providing protection to bony prominences and absorbing drainage. Different products require different wrapping methods, spiral or figure-8. The skin is usually lubricated to prevent drying. These are used for both ambulatory and non-ambulatory patients. The dressing must be applied by a professional and changed 1-2 times weekly. Layered wraps are frequently used for early treatments. Some wraps have visual pressure indicators.
- **Single-layer wraps** (SurePress) are long reusable elastic wraps that are used for early treatment or maintenance and can be used by both ambulatory and non-ambulatory patients. Competent caregivers can be taught to apply these dressings, especially those with visual pressure indicators. Because they are reusable, they are more cost effective than single-use dressings.
- **Therapeutic compression stockings** (Jobst, Juzo, Sig-Varis, Medi-Strumpf, Therapress Duo) are used to prevent ulceration in those with varicose veins and stable venous insufficiency after edema is controlled or with existing ulcers when edema recedes. They are contraindicated with lipodermatosclerosis because of the difficulty fitting the stocking. They may be used for both ambulatory and non-ambulatory patients who are able to apply the stockings. The stockings come in many sizes and colors and may extend from the foot to the knee or the groin. The stockings must be fitted properly and have the correct level of compression:
    - **Class 1**: 20-30 mmHg (varicose veins)
    - **Class 2**: 30-40 mmHg (venous ulcers and prevention)
    - **Class 3**: 40-50 mmHg (refractory venous ulcers & lymphedema)
    - **Class 4**: 50-60 mmHg (lymphedema)

Applying 4-Layer Pressure Bandages

The following is the technique for applying a 4-layer pressure bandage:

- Wounds present on the limb are dressed and padded. The limb is then covered with stockinet. Foam padding is applied to bony prominences over the stockinette.
- The first elastic bandage is applied from the base of the toes or fingers up the limb, overlapping the previous turn by 50%, in a clockwise fashion.
- The next layer of elastic bandage is applied over top of the first, with the same 50% overlap, but in a counterclockwise fashion.

The application of the two elastic bandages in the opposite direction to each other ensures smooth even pressure up the limb. Care is taken with both layers not to exert pressure over the bony prominences to minimize damage to the delicate thin layer of skin in these areas. Short or long stretch bandages are used, depending on the amount of exercise and resting pressure desired.

NON-ELASTIC

There are many products and different types of non-elastic static compression therapy:

- **Unna's boot** (ViscoPaste) is a gauze wrap impregnated with zinc oxide, glycerin, or gelatin to provide a supporting compression "boot" to provide support to the calf muscle pump during ambulation, so they are not suitable for non-ambulatory patients. They can be used for those with peripheral arterial disease. The bandage must be applied carefully without tension. It may be left open to dry or covered with an elastic or self-adherent wrap. The dressings are changed according to the individual needs, determined by a decrease in edema, the amount of exudate, and hygiene with dressing changes ranging from 2 times weekly to every other week.
- **Short-stretch wrap** (Comprilan) is reusable and indicated for ambulatory patients and those with borderline ABIs (0.5-0.8). It is used for both initial and maintenance therapy. Caregivers can be taught to apply, but dressings slip out of place easily.

SHORT STRETCH AND LONG STRETCH BANDAGES

Differences between short and long stretch bandages:

- Short stretch bandages have less elasticity than long stretch. They stretch to 90% of their length whereas long stretch bandages stretch to about 140% of their length.
- Short stretch bandaging exerts more pressure on the limb during ambulation or exercise and low pressure when the limb is at rest. Long stretch bandages exert a higher pressure than short stretch. Since they stretch more, there is less pressure on the limb during exercise than with short stretch. There is more pressure on the limb when at rest, however. This makes it more likely that the long stretch bandage will exert too much pressure during rest, reducing perfusion to tissues and increasing the risk of tissue ischemia.
- Both short and long stretch bandages are applied by exerting tension on the bandage. The amount of tension determines the amount of pressure of the wrapped bandage. Bandaging should never cause numbness or tingling of the distal extremity and circulation, motion, and sensation (CMS) should be frequently monitored while bandages are worn.

NON-ELASTIC ORTHOTICS

Non-elastic orthotics, such as The CircAid Thera-Boot, are stockings with multiple Velcro straps that can be adjusted to fit each patient. The straps make adjusting easy for patients or caregivers. The ankle-foot wrap is attached to cover the foot and ankle but is thin enough to fit into a standard shoe. The orthotic provides continuous compression as well as supporting the calf muscle pump function. The orthotic comes in three sizes (small, medium, and large) according to ankle and calf measurement. It is washable, reusable, and can adjust to changes in limb size, so it is more cost-effective than some other devices. Also, it can be adjusted as needed during activities. The CircAid Thera-Boot was designed specifically for treatment of venous ulcers, but should not be used until edema has subsided. It can be used initially for treatment as well as for maintenance.

INTERMITTENT PNEUMATIC COMPRESSION THERAPY

Intermittent pneumatic compression (IPC) therapy is indicated if static compression therapy is ineffective or if the patient is immobile. (Medicare reimbursement requires a six-month trial of static compression therapy.) IPC devices are used on the lower leg or plantar area of the foot. IPC devices have a garment and a pneumatic pump that inflates the garment. The device for the leg typically has a double-lined stocking that fits over the leg. One lining contains an air bladder with segments so that the intermittent inflations occur segmentally up the leg, increasing venous return. The foot pump takes advantage of the physiologic pumping function in the sole of the foot to stimulate blood flow. The Circulator Boot is an end-diastolic IPC that is timed to the end of diastole to improve arterial flow while improving venous return. Treatments are usually 1-2 times daily for 1-2 hours and decrease edema and promote healing of ulcers. IPC therapy is contraindicated for those with uncompensated heart failure and for those with an active thrombus.

Dressings

Basic Dressing Requirements

The **basic dressing requirements**, regardless of the type, are the following:

- Maintain a moist environment in order to promote healing.
- Absorb wound drainage and prevent leakage.
- Increase wound temperature to promote healing.
- Provide a protective barrier to prevent mechanical injury to the wound.
- Provide a protective barrier to prevent colonization and infection with microorganisms.
- Allow exchange of gases and fluids.
- Retain and absorb odor of the wound or drainage.
- Remove easily without causing additional trauma to the wound or disrupting the healing process.
- Debride wound of dead tissue and exudate.
- Provide protection without toxicity or causing sensitivity reactions.
- Provide a sterile protective covering for the wound.

The dressing that directly covers the wound may be inadequate to absorb large amounts of drainage, so sometimes additional secondary dressings are needed.

Wound Dressing Selection

The proper **dressing** for a wound may change over time depending on wound characteristics:

- The wound environment's moisture content may call for a dressing that either wicks away too much moisture or provides moisture to a dry wound to enhance epithelialization.
- Slough and dry eschar calls for a dressing that will enhance debriding.
- The presence of tunneling or undermining will require a packing material.
- Some wounds need dressings that are absorbent and deodorizing to control exudate.
- Control and prevention of infection is important in some wounds.
- Dressings must allow oxygen, water, and carbon dioxide to be exchanged between the environment and the wound.
- Dressings need to provide warmth as well.
- Dressings must not adhere to or harm the wound tissues but must be kept in place reliably without harming the skin around the wound.

Categories of Dressings and Methods of Securing Dressings

Dressings are considered primary if they are next to the wound surface and secondary if they are used to cover the primary or to secure the dressing. There are **three main types of dressings** to consider when determining which will be the most effective for a particular type of wound:

- **Traditional topical dressings** are used primarily to cover the wound, such as gauze and tulle.
- **Interactive dressings**, such as polymeric films, are generally transparent so that the wound can be observed and are permeable to water vapor and oxygen but provide an effective barrier for microorganisms, such as hyaluronic acid, hydrogel, and foam dressings.
- **Bioactive dressings** provide substances that directly promote wound healing, such as hydrocolloids, alginates, collagens, and chitosan.

Securing a dressing depends on the health of the surrounding skin and the type of dressing. Skin protection and tape may be appropriate. Some are self-adherent. Tubular dressings or wraps can help to secure dressings with fragile skin.

GAUZE DRESSINGS

Gauze dressings are made from cotton, rayon, or polyester, and are frequently used with primary closure where there is little or no exudate. The purpose of these dressings is to provide protection of the partial or full-thickness wounds or those with cavities or tracts. They may be sterile or non-sterile. In the past they were used for wet to dry dressings. Wet-to-dry dressings have little use in current wound care unless the wound is very small because the gauze adheres to the wound and can disrupt granulation or epithelization. Wet to moist saline gauze dressings are sometimes used to treat wounds but are less effective than hydrocolloid dressings. Gauze dressings may be used as secondary dressings with another type of dressing in direct contact with the wound or as packing to fill dead space in combination with amorphous hydrogel or other dressings. When used to fill space, the gauze should be fluffed to avoid causing excess pressure.

TULLE OR IMPREGNATED GAUZE DRESSINGS

Tulle dressings, also known as paraffin gauze, (Jelonet, Paranet) are open weave gauze that are coated with paraffin so they do not adhere to the wound. They are suitable only for flat or shallow wounds. They may be useful for people with sensitive skin. When these are placed in contact with the wound, secondary dressings may be used to absorb exudate.

Impregnated gauze may contain antimicrobials, medications, nutrients, and moisture (such as normal saline). Commonly used gauzes are impregnated with petrolatum, zinc oxide, and iodoform. They are used for partial or full-thickness wounds or those with cavities, tracts, or infection. The choice of gauze depends upon the needs of the wound. They should be loosely packed into cavities and avoid contact with intact skin as they may cause maceration because of the moisture content of the dressing. Exudate should be carefully monitored so dressings can be changed as needed.

FOAM DRESSINGS

Foam dressings are made of semi-permeable hydrophilic foam, and sheet forms may have an impermeable barrier. They come in a wide variety of sizes and shapes (wafers, rolls, pillows, films) depending upon the manufacturer. Some types have a charcoal layer to control odor. Foam dressings provide a warm, moist environment and provide cushioning. Foam dressings may be used for partial and full-thickness wounds. Non-sheet forms are used as packing and are appropriate for minimal to heavy exudate. When used as packing, a secondary non-occlusive dressing is secured over the foam. They are used for leg ulcers as well as pressure injuries. Because they are intended for wounds with exudate in order to provide the appropriate environment for healing, they are not suitable for dry epithelializing wounds or those with eschar. Sheet forms can be used as secondary dressings with alginates, pastes, or powders. Some have adhesive borders. Foam dressings are changed every 2-7 days, depending on the dressing type and the wound.

SEMI-PERMEABLE FILM DRESSINGS

Semi-permeable film (OpSite, Tegaderm, Polyskin II) dressings are composed of polyurethane with a coating of acrylic adhesive so the dressing will adhere to the skin. These types of dressings are frequently used over intravenous sites to allow observation of tissue. They are suitable only for shallow partial-thickness wounds that have little or no exudate because they are not able to absorb; therefore, they are not suitable for infected wounds. They are permeable to air and water vapor but provide a barrier to pathogenic agents and liquid. The tissue under the dressing is maintained in a warm moist environment, encouraging autolysis. The dressings are comfortable and may be left in place for up to 1 week although some people may develop local irritation from the adhesive. Semi-permeable film may be used as a protective dressing and is often used for stage I and II pressure injuries.

Alginates or Other Fiber Gelling Dressings

Alginates (AlgiSite M, Sorbsan, Aquacel, Hydrofiber) are very absorbent dressings made from brown seaweed. Through ion exchange, they absorb drainage and form a hydrophilic gel that conforms to the size and shape of the wound. They are useful for full-thickness wounds with moderate to heavy exudate or slough, such as pressure injuries and cavity wounds, especially if there is undermining or tunneling. They are effective for infected and foul-smelling wounds. Alginates are sold in sheet form or fibers for packing. Alginate dressings or packing fibers are loosely packed into the wound to allow for swelling and then secured with a secondary dressing. They are usually changed once daily. Alginates serve to cushion and protect the wound as well as contain exudate. They are easier to remove than gauze dressings used for packing and cause less discomfort. Alginates need differing times to gel with some requiring 24 hours, so they are not interchangeable.

Hydrocolloid Dressings

Hydrocolloids (DuoDerm, Restore, Tegasorb) are sheets or wafers of absorbent adherent material with an occlusive coating so that they provide a barrier to moisture. They are used for clean granulating wounds that are partial and full thickness with minimal to moderate amounts of drainage. They may be used with pastes or alginates. Hydrocolloids come in various sizes and shapes and can be cut to fit, overlapping the wound by 2-3 cm. They are usually changed about every 2-5 days. Hydrocolloid material may be stiff and should be warmed between the hands to soften before application. Some hydrocolloids emit an unpleasant odor when active. Because the dressings are occlusive, infected wounds should be observed carefully for signs of infection with anaerobic bacteria. They may be used with compression for venous ulcers but are not recommended for third degree burns. Hydrocolloids may cause hypergranulation tissue to form.

Hydrogel Dressings

Hydrogel dressings (AquaForm, Curasol, Hypergel, Elastogel, Vigilon, Intrasite gel) are produced in amorphous form, supplied in tubes, or impregnated in packing strip materials. They are also produced in sheet form, with or without an adhesive border. They have a high moisture content with water or glycerin with hydrophilic sites allowing them to absorb exudate and provide a warm, moist wound environment. Hydrogels are used for partial and full-thickness wounds, dry to small amounts of exudate, necrotic wounds, and infected wounds. They are applied directly to the wound and provide rehydration and autolysis, effectively and quickly debriding the wound. They are usually used with a secondary dressing, such as gauze or films. Dressings may be changed every 1-3 days, depending upon the type of product used. Hydrogels are contraindicated for wounds with heavy exudate, as the leakage may cause maceration of periwound tissue or candidiasis.

Contact Layer Dressings

Contact layers (Dermanet, Mepitel, Tegapore) are composed of woven polyamide net and may be coated with silicone (Mepitel). They adhere lightly to the wound but have pores that allow exudate to pass through to absorbent secondary dressings. They are particularly useful in wounds in which adherence of dressings to the tissue may pose problems, such as with abrasions, second degree burns, grafts, full-thickness granular wounds, and skin damaged by radiotherapy or steroids. They may be used with negative pressure wound therapy. They protect the wound base but are not recommended for shallow or dry wounds. Usually, the contact layer stays in place for up to a week while the secondary absorbent dressings are changed more often. If exudate is extremely viscous, it may not penetrate the net and can build up beneath the contact layer. Some types of contact layers may need to be kept moistened with normal saline so they don't adhere to the wound base.

Composite Dressings

Composites are combination dressings that are frequently used to secure primary dressings or with other dressings, such as alginates. The material in composites varies from one dressing to another, but usually consists of some type of impermeable exterior barrier to prevent leakage of exudate, an absorptive layer (*not* alginate, foam, hydrocolloid, or hydrogel), a semi-adherent or non-adherent surface for covering the wound, and an adhesive rim to secure the dressing to the periwound tissue. Used alone, they are most suitable for partial or shallow full-thickness wounds but used with other dressings they are suitable for larger wounds with minimal to large amounts of exudate. A paper backing must be removed prior to application. They are usually changed about 3 times a week or more often if needed for wounds with larger amount of exudate.

Absorptive Dressings and Wound Fillers

Absorptive dressings (Surgipad, Tendersorb, ABD pad, Exu-dry) are composed of cellulose, cotton, or rayon fibers. Some have adhesive borders. They are highly absorptive and are intended for wounds that have moderate to heavy drainage. They are changed every 1-2 days.

Wound fillers (Biafine WDE, DuoDerm Sterile Hydroactive Paste, Multidex Maltodextrin Wound Dressing) are composed of starch copolymers in numerous different forms, such as pastes, granules, beads, gels, and powders. They fill dead space in shallow wounds, hydrate, provide a warm, moist environment, and absorb exudate. They soften necrotic tissue and aid debridement. Wound fillers are indicated for partial and shallow full-thickness wounds with minimal to moderate exudate and can be used for both infected wounds and uninfected wounds. They are used with secondary dressings, such as films and hydrocolloids. Wound fillers are not recommended for use in dry, eschar-covered, or tunneled wounds. Dressings are usually changed daily.

Wound Pouches

Wound pouches (Convatec Wound Manager, Hollister Wound Manager) are adapted from ostomy appliances and work in a similar way to contain heavy exudate from fistulas, wounds, drains, and tubes. The pouches provide a skin barrier to protect the skin and a drainage spout so that the pouch can be attached to straight drainage and a bedside bag. The pouch provides odor control as well. The opening in the pouch is cut to fit around the wound and paste, such as Stomahesive, is applied about the cut opening to ensure seal. The skin is usually wiped with a skin barrier prior to application, and any skin crevices are filled with paste. Forceps are used to feed drains or tubes through the opening of the pouch. Pouches are usually changed about every 4-7 days or when there is leakage or drainage under appliance.

Wound Debridement

Autolytic Debridement

Autolysis takes advantage of the body's enzymes and white blood cells to debride the wound by using proteolytic, fibrinolytic, and collagenolytic enzymes to soften and liquefy slough and eschar. Autolysis takes place in a warm, moist environment with adequate vasculature to provide white blood cells and neutrophils, so the neutrophil count must be adequate (>500 mm^3) or sepsis can occur. Autolysis is most successful in stage III or IV uninfected wounds and when exudate is light to moderate so that occlusive dressings can be maintained. Autolysis does not damage the periwound tissue, and it is an easy method of debridement, causing very little discomfort. However, it is slower than some methods, taking 72-96 hours before effects are demonstrated. Autolysis may be combined with other types of debridement, using autolysis first to soften and loosen eschar. Autolysis requires close monitoring of the wound, which may appear to enlarge as the eschar dissolves, showing the true dimensions of the wound.

Procedures and Selection of Agents

Autolytic debridement requires a warm, moist, atmosphere, so occlusive or semi-occlusive dressings must be applied to the wound area. All moisture-retentive dressings promote autolysis to some degree, even when other methods of debridement are used, but as a sole means of debridement, it is recommended only for relatively small, uninfected wounds. The dressings most commonly used for autolytic debridement include:

- **Hydrocolloids** provide absorbency for wounds with small amounts of exudate, but may promote anaerobic infections if the dressing is occlusive.
- **Alginate dressings** provide added absorbency for wounds with large amounts of exudate, but require a secondary dressing to secure them.
- **Hydrogels** are particularly helpful when wounds are dry because they add necessary moisture and promote rapid autolysis.
- **Transparent films** promote autolysis for very small, shallow wounds or when used as a secondary dressing.

As the wound debrides, odor and drainage increase, so periwound tissue must be protected from exudate.

Enzymatic Debridement

Enzymatic debridement is a method of chemical debridement that can be used on any type of wound that has a large amount of necrosis and eschar, especially chronic wounds and burns. Enzymes either directly digest the fibrin, bacteria, leukocytes, and other cell debris that comprises slough or dissolves the collagen that secures it to the wound. Enzymes need a moist environment, so if enzymes are used to debride dry eschar, the eschar must be crosshatched through the upper layers with a scalpel to allow the enzymes to penetrate the eschar. Enzymes are selective and do not damage viable tissue although some people have local irritation from the enzymes, particularly if the enzyme contains papain. Enzymatic debridement is relatively fast-acting but can still take days to weeks to complete debridement, especially with large wounds, so it is slower than some other techniques.

Procedures and Selection of Agents

Enzymatic debridement uses chemical enzymes. Enzymes can be used with any type of dressing, but the enzymes need to be applied to necrotic tissue 1-2 times daily, so long-term dressings are not cost-effective. Moisture-retentive dressings speed debridement. Two types of enzyme preparations are used:

- **Collagenase** (Santyl), derived from *Clostridium* bacteria, digests denatured collagen and is administered once daily by tongue blade into deep wounds or applied to gauze for shallow wounds. It is inactivated by low pH (optimum range is 6-8) hexachlorophene and heavy metal ions, including mercury, zinc, silver, and Burow's solution.
- **Papain/urea** combinations (Accuzyme, Panafil White, Panafil, Gladase), derived from papaya, with or without chlorophyllin copper complex sodium, which reduces inflammation and odor. This enzyme digests nonviable protein composing the necrotic tissue. It is applied 1-2 times daily and is inactivated by hydrogen peroxide and salts of heavy metals, including lead, silver, and mercury. It works at a pH of 3-12.

Biological Debridement with Maggots

Maggot debridement is inexpensive, faster than other non-surgical therapies, and effective, but it is usually saved for cases not responding well to other therapy. Sterilized maggots (blowfly larvae) secrete proteolytic enzymes, including collagenase, which debrides the wound, as well as growth factors and cytokines, which increase healing. The teeth of the maggots penetrate the eschar, aiding the enzymes. While the FDA has approved Medical Maggots only for debridement, numerous reports indicate that they also are effective against wound infections, such as MRSA. Antibiotics are often given concurrently with infected wounds because maggots can pick up pathogens in the wound and spread them in the tissue and to the bloodstream. Maggots are effective for many wounds, including pressure and stasis ulcers and burns. Maggots cannot be used with hydrogels. Periwound tissue must be protected from exudate. Large numbers of maggots should not be used in areas where blood vessels are exposed or damaged to prevent bleeding. Those on anticoagulants must be observed for bleeding.

Procedure

Medical Maggots are applied to the open wound. The periwound tissue must be protected. The procedure is as follows:

1. A wound pattern is transferred onto a hydrocolloid pad, the opening is cut, and then the pad applied to the skin with the wound exposed. The pattern is used to cut an opening in a semi-permeable film for an outer dressing.
2. Maggots are wiped from the container with a saline-dampened 2X2 gauze (about 5-10 maggots per cm^2 wound size). The gauze is loosely packed into the wound.
3. A porous mesh (Creature Comfort) is placed over the wound and secured to the hydrocolloid with tape or glue, creating a maggot cage.
4. Transparent film is placed over the hydrocolloid, making sure that the cutout area is over the cage so that the maggots have air and drainage can escape. Saline-dampened gauze is placed loosely over cage.
5. Dry gauze is used for the outer dressing and changed every 4-8 hours as needed.
6. Maggots are wiped from the wound after 48 hours, and the wound is irrigated with normal saline.

Mechanical Debridement

Wet to Dry

Wet-to-dry debridement is a common treatment in use for many years to debride wounds and absorb exudate, but it is non-selective in that it can pull healthy and granulating tissue from wounds as well. Treatment usually involves applying saline-moistened gauze to a wound and allowing it to dry for 4-6 hours and then pulling it off the wound. Using this approach to removing necrotic tissue can take days to weeks, depending upon the extent of the wound. It's important in wet-to-dry debridement that the dressings dry out completely, so the dressing should be moist but not saturated. One major drawback to wet-to-dry debridement is that it is quite painful, but wetting the gauze prior to removal to ease the pain decreases the effectiveness. This method requires frequent dressing changes and careful aseptic technique. Most experts in wound care no longer recommend wet-to-dry debridement or advise it only initially for heavily necrotic wounds.

Sharp Debridement

Sharp (instrumental) debridement involves the cutting away of necrotic tissue using forceps, scissors, and a scalpel. This is the most aggressive form of debridement that can be done by non-physician medical personnel, and regulations about doing this therapy vary from state to state. In some states, it is in the scope of practice for RNs while in other states it is within the scope of physical therapists' duties. Sharp debridement cleans the wound much faster than other non-surgical forms of debridement, promoting faster healing, and is selective as the person doing the debridement controls the type and amount of tissue that is removed. The procedure involves:

1. Using aseptic technique and sterile equipment.
2. Cleansing the site of debridement with an antiseptic.
3. Holding the tissue taut with forceps to establish a plane of dissection.
4. Dissecting carefully, avoiding vasculature.
5. Irrigating the wound with normal saline upon completion.

Surgical Debridement

Surgical debridement is instrumental dissection of necrotic tissue under general, spinal, or local anesthesia. It is most commonly used when very large amounts of tissue must be debrided, such as with extensive burns, or when there is a serious infection and immediate debridement is needed in order to effectively treat the wound infection. General anesthesia allows extensive debridement to be done without the patient suffering associated pain and trauma although postoperative pain is common. One advantage is that most debridement can be done in one procedure. Surgical debridement has been shown to stimulate healing in diabetic ulcers. However, there are risks associated with anesthesia and post-operative wound infections can occur. It is also much more costly than other methods. An alternative surgical method is **laser debridement**, which can cut away necrotic tissue. Pulsed laser beams are less damaging to adjacent tissue than continuous lasers.

Chemical Cauterization

Chemical cauterization with silver nitrate is sometimes used to treat hypergranulation. Cauterization uses heat to burn or sear abnormal cells in order to destroy them. Silver nitrate sticks are wet with water to activate and are then gently rolled over the tissue to be treated for a short time. Chemical cauterization is used infrequently, for such things as treatment of nosebleeds and warts. The most common uses for chemical cauterization in wounds or skin lesions are to control hypergranulation tissue that grows in wounds, especially about stomas or to treat warts. Hypergranulation is excessive soft flaccid granulating tissue that is raised above the level of the periwound tissue, preventing proper epithelization, and it may reflect excess moisture in the wound. Hypergranulation tissue is often friable and bleeds easily. It may produce both exudates that interfere with healing and odor. Treatment may be repeated 2 times daily for 1-4 days until excess tissue sloughs.

Topical Agents

Topical Antibiotics

Topical antibiotics may be used to treat localized wound infections based on results of culture and sensitivities so that the treatment is appropriate for the invading microorganism. Topical antibiotics include:

- **Cadexomer Iodine** (Iodosorb) is an iodine preparation formulated to be less toxic to granulating tissue. It can be applied as a powder, paste, or ointment. The ointment contains beads with iodine. The beads swell in contact with exudate, slowly releasing the iodine, which is affective against a broad range of bacteria, such as *Staphylococcus aureus, MRSA, Streptococcus, and Pseudomonas,* as well as viruses and fungi.
- **Gentamicin sulfate**, prepared as a cream or ointment, is a broad-spectrum antibiotic that is effective against both primary and secondary skin infections in stasis and other injuries or skin lesions. It is bactericidal against *Staphylococcus aureus, Streptococcus, and Pseudomonas,* but does not have antiviral or antifungal properties.
- **Metronidazole**, prepared as a gel or a wax-glycerin cream, is effective against MRSA infections.
- **Mupirocin 2%**, prepared in an ointment, is effective primarily against Gram-positive bacteria and is used primarily for *Staphylococcus, MRSA,* and *Streptococcus.* It is frequently used to treat nasal colonization of *Staphylococcus* because colonization is implicated in subsequent wound infections.
- **Polymyxin B sulfate-Bacitracin zinc-neomycin ointment** (Neosporin) is frequently used to prevent infections in small cuts and lacerations, but it can also be used in infected wounds and is active against *Staphylococcus aureus, Streptococcus and Pseudomonas.*
- **Polymyxin B sulfate-Gramicidin cream** is similar to that above except it is also effective against *MRSA.*
- **Silver sulfadiazine** (2-7%) is frequently used in burn treatment and has a strong antimicrobial action against *Staphylococcus aureus, MRSA, Streptococcus, and Pseudomonas.*
- **Silver (ionized)**, prepared in absorbent sheets and activated with sterile water, is effective against the same organisms as silver sulfadiazine. The moist environment increases re-epithelialization.

Regranex Gel to Stimulate Wound Healing

Regranex gel contains becaplermin, which is a recombinant human platelet-derived growth factor (Rh-PDGF). Regranex causes gathering and replication of cells to heal the wound and encourages granulation. Regranex gel is indicated for deep diabetic neuropathic ulcers, extending into or below subcutaneous tissue. It has not been studied for use with superficial diabetic ulcers or pressure injuries. The wound must have a good blood supply for the gel to be effective. The wound must also be debrided, infection must be controlled, pressure must be relieved, and the wound bed must stay moist for the best outcome. The wound should show improved healing within 10 weeks and be healed within 5 months. It should not be used if cancer is present at the site of the wound, sutures or staples are present, or if joints, ligaments, or tendons are exposed.

Topical Agents for Peri-Wound Skin Protection

Moisture Barrier Paste

Moisture barrier pastes are ointments with powder added to improve absorption and make them more durable and solid, providing a thick skin barrier. Many are zinc oxide based, making them somewhat difficult to remove. Mineral oil is often used to remove the paste. Some paste products now on the market are transparent so that the skin underneath can be monitored. Additionally, some pastes contain karaya or carboxymethyl cellulose to increase adherence to the tissue. Pastes are frequently used over denuded or excoriated tissue to absorb exudate and protect from drainage, urine, or feces, so they are used for both peri-anal and peri-wound tissues. While pastes are more resistant to drainage than ointments and adhere better to denuded skin, they do interfere with adhesion of dressings, and zinc oxide cannot be used with some wound care treatments. Pastes are usually reapplied with each dressing change without being completely removed first. Some **barrier pastes** include:

- Critic-Aid Skin Paste
- Ilex Skin Protectant Paste
- Remedy Calazime Protectant Paste

Moisture Barrier Ointment

Moisture barrier ointments provide protection for the skin from moisture, exudate, urine, and feces with petrolatum or zinc oxide based-products packaged in tubes or small individual packets. These products, because of their greasy nature, can interfere with adhesion of the wound dressings, and some wound care products cannot be used with zinc oxide, so they have limited application. This type of barrier is frequently used with patients who are incontinent to prevent incontinence dermatitis, which can deteriorate into pressure injuries. Barrier ointments are usually reapplied with each dressing or adult brief change, so overall costs may be higher than with barrier films that can be applied less frequently. Some products contain karaya or carboxymethyl cellulose (hydrophilics) to improve adherence to the skin. Some **barrier ointment products** include:

- Calmoseptine Ointment
- Lantiseptic Skin Protectant
- Proshield Plus Skin Protectant
- Critic-Aid Clear Hydrophilic Ointment

Skin Sealants

While a warm, moist environment is optimum for wound healing, the exudate poses a risk to adjacent tissue, which must be protected or it will macerate, potentially ulcerating and increasing the size of the wound. Various topical agents are used to protect peri-wound skin, including skin sealants, which are film-forming barriers composed of a polymer in a fast-drying solvent, applied every 1-4 days, depending on the product. When the sealant is applied to the skin, the solvent (often isopropyl alcohol) dissolves, leaving the transparent plasticized polymer barrier over the tissue. It may be applied to intact or irritated tissue although there may be some discomfort from the alcohol solvent with broken skin. Sealants can be used to protect skin from exudate, urine, stool, chemicals, and adhesive stripping. Sealants are applied with wipes, wands, or sprays. Some **sealant products** include:

- Skin Prep
- Shield Skin
- Bard Protective Barrier Film Wipe
- Allkare Convatec
- Cavilon No Sting Barrier Film (does not use alcohol)

Skin Barrier Powders

Skin barrier powders are used as an initial barrier on denuded skin to provide an adherent base for ointments, pastes, or solid skin adhesive barriers. The powder is sprinkled over the denuded area, and excess is removed before application of the second barrier. Powders should be applied thinly because excess will impair adhesion of other barrier products, and they should not be used on intact skin, as they will not properly adhere. Skin barrier powders contain powder pectin, karaya, gelatine, carboxymethyl cellulose or combinations. They are frequently used with ostomy products when the skin has become weepy. Warm moist areas are ideal for fungus growth, which causes burning and itching, so the addition of antifungal powder may be necessary as well to promote healing. Use of the skin barrier powders should be discontinued as soon as the skin heals. **Skin barrier powders** include:

- Stomahesive Protective Powder
- Karaya Powder
- Premium Powder

Solid Skin Barriers

Solid skin barriers are solid waterproof moldable adhesive skin barriers, usually in the form of rings, strips, or wafers that provide skin protection for moisture, exudate, urine, or feces. They may contain hydrocolloids, pectin, karaya, gelatine, carboxymethyl cellulose or combinations. They are frequently used with urostomies and ileostomies as a base to anchor appliances and protect the skin from discharge. They may be cut to fit snugly around wounds. While they are frequently left in place for days at a time, it is possible for drainage to leak under the barrier, so they must be checked. Some swell when in contact with discharge and have acidic pH to discourage growth of organisms. Solid skin barriers are more durable than ointments or pastes, but they must be removed carefully to prevent stripping of the skin, especially if they are applied in an area that receives pressure, such as the coccyx. **Solid skin barriers** include:

- Hollister Flextend
- Stomahesive
- Eakin
- Premium Skin Barrier

Skin Transfer and Surgical Closure

Skin Substitutes

Tissue engineered skin and skin substitutes have been developed in spite of tremendous difficulties in the creation of non-contaminated cell cultures and the transport of these cells to operating rooms when they are needed. They are applied after the wound has been debrided:

- **Apligraf** is made of a bovine collagen mesh with living neonatal fibroblasts from neonatal foreskin. When applied, it looks like a mesh, and then it changes to a gel after about 7 days. It is a "living skin equivalent" that provides growth factors to the wound to stimulate healing. Apligraf is transported on media in a petri dish and must be kept warm until it is used. It is placed over a wound free from necrotic material and infection before a compression dressing is applied.
- **Dermagraft** is a cryopreserved skin substitute that also uses neonatal fibroblasts from neonatal foreskin but without the bovine material. It is used for diabetic foot ulcers.

Skin Flaps

A skin flap may be used to repair a wound that has a poor vascular supply. A section of skin is cut, leaving one end of the flap attached to its original site. The flap is then brought forward or twisted on its axis to reach the wound site. Some flaps are sutured to more distant sites, such as the arm to the face. The free end of the flap is sutured into the wound. When this end of the flap grows into the wound and new blood vessels are generated to support it, the other end of the flap is cut away from the donor site. The donor site is sutured or grafted. Sometimes the skin is stretched by the placement or injection of tissue expanders prior to raising the flap to increase the amount of skin available.

Skin Grafts

Skin grafts speed healing and reduce fluid loss from burns and wounds. They enhance the wound cosmetically. Grafts may be taken from the patient's body (autograft), or from a cadaver (allograft). Skin substitutes (Apligraf or Dermagraft) or animal tissue, such as from a pig (xenograft), may also be used. Xenografts last 3-5 days before rejection and are used for partial wound healing and protection prior to permanent grafting with an autograft or allograft. Skin grafts may be partial or split thickness (epidermis and part of dermal layer) or full thickness (epidermis and entire dermis):

- **Partial thickness grafts** may not regain sebaceous or sweat glands, causing the area to be dry and to be warmer than the rest of the body. Hair follicles and nerves may regenerate in grafted areas.
- **Full thickness grafts** rely on neovascularization to stay vital and to grow into the defect. They provide the most natural appearance but can be used only in small areas, unlike a split thickness graft.

Staples

Staples may be used to close superficial wounds of the scalp, neck, axillae, extremities, trunk, or external genitalia. The procedure is as follows:

1. Position the patient so that the wound is easily accessed.
2. Irrigate the wound with NS, using a 10-mL syringe with an 18-gauge needle.
3. Wipe the skin in a 7-8 cm diameter area about the wound with an antiseptic.
4. Apply gloves and administer local anesthetic, typically 1% or 2% lidocaine.
5. Bring the skin edges together and place the stapling device over the edges, holding it perpendicular to the skin and depressing the lever.
6. Continue placing staples about every quarter inch.
7. Apply topical antibiotic ointment and dressing.

Staples should be removed within 7-10 days for staples in the limbs, hands, feet, and trunk, in 3-5 days for the face/neck, and 5-7 days for the ear or scalp as prolonged staple closure may result in scarring and increased risk of infection.

Sutures

Sutures are used for superficial wounds of the scalp, face, nose, lips, mucous membranes, neck, axillae, trunk, extremities, and external genitalia, for superficial dehiscence, and for intermediate repairs with layer closures. The healthcare provider should determine the appropriate needle, suture material, and suturing technique. Procedure:

1. Position patient so that the wound is easily accessed.
2. Apply povidone-iodine with swab from wound edges outward to a circle of at least 4 cm beyond the wound on all sides.
3. Apply gloves and administer local anesthetic (usually lidocaine 1% or 2% with or without epinephrine).
4. Irrigate the wound with normal saline (60-100 mL NS), trim ragged edges with sterile scissors, undermine the edges if necessary to assure approximation.
5. Hold needle holder with suture in dominant hand and toothed forceps in the other to grasp the edges of the wound, and begin suturing with sutures about 0.5 cm from the wound edge.
6. Cleanse the suture line with NS and apply dry dressing.
7. Advise the patient of the length of time the sutures must remain in place.

Prior to suture removal, if the sutures are crusted, cleanse with a cotton-tipped applicator and hydrogen peroxide, remove hydrogen peroxide with applicator saturated with NS, and then dry with gauze.

Surgical/Vascular Interventions for Arterial Insufficiency/Ulcers

The goals of management for arterial insufficiency and ulcers are to improve perfusion and save the limb, but lifestyle changes and medications may be insufficient. There are a number of indications for surgical intervention:

- Poor healing prognosis includes those with ABI <0.5 because their perfusion is severely compromised.
- Failure to respond to conservative treatment (medications and lifestyle changes) even with an ABI >0.5.
- Intolerable pain, such as with severe intermittent claudication, which is incapacitating and limits the patient's ability to work or carry out activities. Rest pain is an indication that medical treatment is insufficient.
- Limb-threatening condition, such as severe ischemia with increasing pain at rest, infection, and/or gangrene. Infection can cause a wound to deteriorate rapidly.
- Surgical intervention is indicated only for those patients with patent distal vessels as demonstrated by radiologic imaging procedures.

Surgical/Vascular Interventions for Severe Arterial Insufficiency

Surgical/vascular interventions for treatment of severe arterial insufficiency include 3 different types of procedures:

- **Bypass grafts** in which a section of the saphenous vein or an upper extremity vein are harvested to use to bypass damaged arteries and supply blood to distal vessels. Because veins have valves, they must be reversed or stripped of valves prior to attachment. Synthetic grafts are also sometimes used, but they have a much higher failure rate.
- **Angioplasty** can be used if disease is not extensive (>10 in length), but arteries must be large enough to accommodate the procedure safely. Initial results are good but long-term rates have been less positive although the use of anticoagulants improves success rates.
- **Amputation** is the procedure that treatment tries to avoid, but it is sometimes required if ischemia is irreversible or if there is severe necrosis and infection that is life threatening.

Additional Wound Therapy Options

Negative Pressure Wound Therapy

Negative pressure wound therapy (NPWT) uses subatmospheric (negative) pressure with a suction unit and a semi-occlusive vapor-permeable dressing. The suction reduces periwound and interstitial edema, decompressing vessels and improving circulation. It also stimulates production of new cells and decreases colonization of bacteria. NPWT also increases the rate of granulation and re-epithelialization so that wounds heal more quickly. The wound must be debrided of necrotic tissue prior to treatment. NPWT is used for a variety of difficult to heal wounds, especially those that show less than 30% healing in 4 weeks of post-debridement treatment or those with excessive exudate, including the following:

- Chronic stage II and IV pressure injuries
- Skin flaps
- Diabetic ulcers
- Acute wounds
- Burns, both partial and full-thickness
- Unresponsive arterial and venous ulcers
- Surgical wounds and those with dehiscence

It is **contraindicated** in the below conditions:

- Wound malignancy
- Untreated osteomyelitis
- Exposed blood vessels or organs
- Nonenteric, unexplored fistulas

Application

Application of negative pressure wound therapy is done after the wound is determined to be appropriate for this treatment and debridement is completed, leaving the wound tissue exposed. There are a number of different electrical suction NPWT systems, such as the VAC (vacuum-assisted closure) system and the Versatile Implant (VI). Application steps include:

1. Apply nonadherent porous foam cut to fit, and completely cover the wound.
   a. **Polyurethane** (hydrophobic, repelling moisture) is used for all wounds EXCEPT those that are painful or have tunneling or sinus tracts, deep trauma wounds, and wounds needing controlled growth of granulation.
   b. **Polyvinyl** (hydrophilic), is used for all wounds EXCEPT deep wounds with moderate granulation or flaps and deep pressure injuries.
2. Secure foam occlusive transparent film.
3. Cut opening to accommodate the drainage tube in the dressing and attach drainage tube.
4. Attach tube to suction canister, creating closed system.
5. Set pressure to 75-125, as indicated.
6. Change dressings 2-3 times weekly.

Hyperbaric Oxygen Treatments

Hyperbaric oxygen therapy (HBOT) is treatment in a high-pressure chamber while breathing 100% oxygen, which increases available oxygen to tissues by 10-20 times. Blood that is saturated increases perfusion of the tissues. HBOT has shown considerable promise in reducing the need for amputation resulting from ulcerations of the lower extremities, but it is critical that treatment be instituted early enough while the potential for salvage remains. HBOT is used for a number of conditions, but is especially important for hypoxic wounds, such as those associated with peripheral arterial insufficiency, compromised skin from grafts, and diabetic ulcers. Treatment protocols vary according to the type of wound, but are limited to 90 minutes to avoid oxygen toxicity. HBOT has the following effects:

- Hyperoxygenation of blood and tissue
- Vasoconstriction, reducing capillary leakage
- Angiogenesis because of increased fibroblasts and collagen
- Increased antibiotic effectiveness for those needing active transport across cell walls (fluoroquinolone, amphotericin B, aminoglycosides)

Hyperbaric oxygen therapy (HBOT) supplies oxygen at pressures of 2-3 times that of the atmosphere. The patient is treated in a multi-person or single person chamber. This therapy is delivered by specially trained physicians since oxygen toxicity side effects are possible. Transcutaneous oximetry levels should reach >200 mmHg for HBOT to be effective. One or two hours of HBOT results in a higher amount of dissolved oxygen in the blood, and it remains for a prolonged period of time. HBOT is used for pressure injuries, burns, gas gangrene, radiation burns, skin grafts and flaps, vascular ulcers, osteomyelitis, and crush injuries.

Biophysical Technologies

Ultraviolet Light

Ultraviolet light B (UVB) can be used to induce inflammation, stimulate granulation, and decompose necrotic tissue. However, Ultraviolet light C (UVC) is the type most often used for wound healing, primarily for its bacteriocidal action, as it is effective against MRSA and other antibiotic-resistant bacteria (destroying 100%) and reduces overall bioburden in infected wounds. Most equipment comes with distance guides that help to ensure proper positioning in relation to the wound:

- Provide eye protection to the patient and the operator to prevent damage to the retina.
- Provide protection to periwound skin by applying petrolatum jelly.
- Position the light the proper distance (one inch) from the wound.
- Provide treatment according to manufacturer's guidelines.

UV light therapy is contraindicated if the patient has sensitive skin, or is taking medications that cause photosensitization such as tetracyclines, sulfonamides, quinolones, amiodarone, quinidine, phenothiazines, psoralens, and others.

Electrical Stimulation

Electrical stimulation (ES) is used to promote healing of a wound, as it stimulates proliferation of epidermal cells and activity of fibroblasts, which produce collagen. ES is most often provided by high voltage pulsed current (HVPC). It uses short pulses of current followed by longer pauses, which stimulates fibroblasts and growth factors. Tissue perfusion is improved with increased blood flow and development of new capillaries, and edema is decreased. ES promotes phagocytosis and has a bacteriocidal effect. It helps to relieve diabetic neuropathic pain. Treatments last 45-60 minutes and are given 5-7 times a week. Precautions include avoiding placement of the electrodes near the heart or larynx. Wounds treated with silver products must be rinsed thoroughly to remove all traces of silver before electrical stimulation is applied.

Water-Filtered Infrared-A Therapy

Water-filtered infrared-A (wIRA) uses heat radiation to help acute and chronic wounds heal. The infrared halogen light is filtered with water to increase humidity and prevent it from heating only the skin surface, causing skin irritation. Water-filtered infrared-A therapy acts by increasing the temperature in the wound, thereby increasing oxygen partial pressure and perfusion and thus the energy supply to the tissues. This treatment can be particularly useful in large wounds in which the center of the wound is hypoxic and has a positive effect on the amount of pain caused by the wound. The wIRA radiator does not contact the skin, the therapy is easily performed, and it is pain-free for the patient. It can be used on wound seromas and pressure injuries with good effect.

Pharmacologic Measures to Maximize Perfusion

The primary focus of pharmacologic measures to maximize perfusion is to reduce the risk of thromboses:

- **Antiplatelet agents** such as aspirin, Ticlid, and Plavix interfere with the function of the plasma membrane, interfering with clotting. These agents are ineffective to treat clots but prevent clot formation.
- **Vasodilators** may divert blood from ischemic areas, but some may be indicated, such as Pietal, which dilates arteries, decreases clotting, and is used for control of intermittent claudication.
- **Antilipemics** such as Zocor and Questran, slow progression of atherosclerosis.
- **Hemorheologics**, such as Trental, reduce fibrinogen, reducing blood viscosity and rigidity of erythrocytes; however, clinical studies show limited benefit. It may be used for intermittent claudication.
- **Analgesics** may be necessary to improve quality of life. Opioids may be needed in some cases.

- **Thrombolytics** may be injected into a blocked artery under angiography to dissolve clots.
- **Anticoagulants**, such as Coumadin and Lovenox, prevent blood clots from forming.

Review Video: Antiplatelets and Thrombolytics
Visit mometrix.com/academy and enter code: 711284

Growth Factor Treatments

Growth factors are proteins that are necessary for growth and migration of cells, and are thus critical elements in healing of wounds. Growth factors may be isolated from tumor cells, platelets, macrophages, ovarian follicles, and the placenta. Recombinant DNA techniques have allowed production of synthetic growth factor from bacterial cultures or human cells with the growth factor genes. Growth factors are applied topically to the wound. There are a number of different **types of growth factors** in use or study, including:

- **Connective Tissue Growth Factor (CTGF)** is being studied for use to combat fibrosis.
- **Epidermal Growth Factor (EGF)** is used for burns and venous ulcers.
- **Fibroblast Growth Factor (FGF)** is used for burns and pressure injuries.
- **Insulin-Like Growth Factor (IGF)** is being studied as a means to reduce HbA1c in diabetes.
- **Platelet-Derived Growth Factor (PDGF)** is used for pressure and diabetic ulcers.
- **Transforming Growth Factor-Beta (TGF-β)** is used with chronic skin ulcers.

Leech Therapy

Leech therapy, known medically as hirudotherapy, is the practice of using leeches at the site of wounds to induce vasodilation, minimize coagulation (through the secretion of hirudin in their saliva), and decrease inflammation, thereby promoting wound healing. By maintaining a localized anticoagulated state, blood flow is sustained to the wound, helping to repair the tissue and prevent necrosis. The leeches also drain excess blood, which controls inflammation, another inhibitory mechanism for wound healing. Before considering leech therapy for wound healing or management of chronic wounds, active infection must be controlled, and circulation to the wound must be demonstrated. Laboratory work for hematocrit and hemoglobin should be drawn to ensure appropriate blood volume, as blood loss may occur with leech therapy, depending on the duration of the treatment, the surface area of the wound, and the number of leeches used.

Mist Therapy

Mist therapy is an adjunctive therapy for wound healing that is meant to be used in addition to more traditional measures such as cleaning/debriding and dressing changes. This therapy involves the application of a saline-based mist to the wound surface and periwound area that is administered using a low-frequence ultrasound device. This therapy is both non-invasive and painless, which minimizes associated risks. The saline acts to reduce bacteria on and around the wound while stimulating blood flow to the wound, a necessary element of the healing process. Over time, the saline can also act as a mild debriding agent by removing necrotic tissue that is within the wound bed or margins.

Patient Comfort

Wound Care Environment During Wound Treatment

The wound care environment is important, especially when wound treatment is painful. The room should be clean, quiet, non-stressful, comfortably warm, and appropriately lighted. Privacy must be insured, and there should be no interruptions:

1. Explain the procedure to the patient.
2. Consider the need for another person to hold the patient's hand during the procedure.
3. Enlist help to minimize the time needed for the treatment.
4. Uncover only the area of the body with the wound.
5. Do not expose the wound until all preparations have been made and treatment is ready to begin.
6. Treat the wound as gently as possible and as little as possible to minimize pain.
7. Allow time-outs as needed to keep the patient comfortable.
8. Allow space in which to perform the procedure so that the wound is not accidentally bumped.
9. Check with the patient frequently during the treatment and allow breaks as needed for repositioning or relief from pain or stress.

Patient Comfort During Wound Treatment

Wound treatments may be very uncomfortable for the patient, so proper **premedication with analgesics** is important:

- Work with the patient to schedule the treatment for an appropriate time.
- Help the patient to use the restroom prior to treatment.
- Position the patient so that all parts of the body are supported, allowing the patient to relax as much as possible. Comfort will allow the patient to maintain the position that allows optimal access to the wound for as long as is necessary.
- Take time to check that the patient is comfortable and without pain before beginning the procedure.
- Check to see that breathing is unimpaired if the patient is lying prone. Small adjustments in position are important.

Removing a Dressing

The proper method to remove a dressing is described below:

1. Wash hands and don gloves.
2. Place open bag near the wound so the old dressing can be placed directly into the bag without leaking onto the bed linens or nearby surfaces.
3. Open plastic bag and fold top down so that only the interior of the bag is exposed.
4. Remove adhesive dressing slowly. Rapid removal can tear the top layer from periwound skin and from the wound bed. Dressings that are adherent should be soaked until easy removal is obtained. The use of chemical adhesive removers can cause the remover to leak into the wound, causing pain and destruction of newly formed tissues.
5. Place the dressing into the bag, remove the gloves, and put them into the bag also. Never reuse top layers of a dressing.
6. Grasp the bag by the outside and tie a knot in it.
7. Place it into a biohazard waste container.
8. Wash hands and don clean gloves to continue working with the wound.

Pain Management

Considerations Regarding Pain Control Measures

Good wound care must include the assessment and management of pain. Dressing changes, especially, are often very painful. There are a number of considerations:

- Pain assessment should be done regularly, allowing the patient to describe the type and extent of pain as well as the patient's response to analgesia in order to manage pain optimally.
- Poor perfusion and infection increase pain, so measures should aim at increasing circulation/oxygenation of the wound, assessing for signs of infection, and instituting treatment.
- Increasing fluid intake and providing proper nutrition improve wound condition and reduce pain.
- Pain medications should be given as needed and prior to dressing changes. With severe pain, such as burns, patient-controlled analgesia (PCA) devices help the patient feel more independent and relieve fear of pain. Medications to relieve anxiety may potentiate pain medications.
- Fungating cancerous lesions may require modifications in dressing routines to decrease dressing changes and periwound care to prevent painful maceration.

Interventions for Non-Cyclic, Cyclic, and Persistent Wound Pain

Non-cyclic pain occurs in specific non-routine situations, such as with periodic wound debridement. The patient should be provided pain medication prior to the treatment, and other pain relief methods, such as topical anesthetics may be considered. Surgical or sharp debridement may be avoided or decreased by using hydrogel, hydrocolloids, enzymatic agents, hypertonic saline, or transparent dressings.

Cyclic pain is predictable pain that occurs in a regular cycle, such as with daily changing of dressings. Pain should be managed with regular pain medications, and other methods of reducing pain may include using dressings that are less painful (avoiding wet to dry), scheduling wound care when the patient is not fatigued, soaking dressing before removal, keeping the wound bed moist, limiting packing, relieving pressure, taking time outs during procedures, and providing comfortable positioning.

Persistent wound pain requires regularly-scheduled pain control as well as other pain-reducing methods, such as relaxation and electrical nerve stimulation (EMS). The area may be splinted to decrease pressure. Antibiotics may be used to reduce infection.

Pharmacologic Treatment of Wound Pain

Topical Anesthetics

There are numerous different types of pain medications that may be used to control pain from wounds, including **topical anesthetics**:

- **Lidocaine 2-4%** is frequently used during debridement or dressing changes. Lidocaine is useful only superficially and may take 15-30 minutes before it is effective.
- **Eutectic Mixture of Local Anesthetics (EMLA Cream)** provides good pain control. The wound is first cleansed, and then the cream is applied thickly (1/4 inch), extending about 1/2 inch past the wound to the peri-wound tissue. The wound is then covered with plastic wrap, which is secured and left in place for about 20 minutes. The wrapped time may be extended to 45-60 minutes if necessary to completely numb the tissue. The tissue should remain numb for about 1 hour after the plastic wrap is removed, allowing time for the wound to be cleansed, debrided, and/or redressed.

Regional Anesthesia

Regional anesthesia (injectable subcutaneous and perineural medications) is administered locally about the wound or as nerve blocks. Medications include lidocaine, bupivacaine and tetracaine in solution. Epinephrine is sometimes added to increase vasoconstriction and reduce bleeding although it is avoided in distal areas of the limbs (hands and feet) to prevent ischemia.

- **Field blockade** involves injecting the anesthetic into the periwound tissue or into the wound margins. The effect may be decreased by inflammation. The effects last for limited periods of time.
- **Regional nerve blocks** may involve single injections, the effects of which are limited in duration but can provide pain relief for treatments. Techniques that use continuous catheter infusions are longer lasting and can be controlled more precisely. Blocks may involve nerves proximal to affected areas, such as peripheral nerve blocks, or large nerve blocks near the spinal cord, such as percutaneous lumbar sympathetic blocks (LSB). Long-term blocks may use alcohol-based medications to permanently inactivate the nerves.

Systemic Medications

Systemic medications may be given orally or by injection into muscles, subcutaneous tissue, or veins. The 3-step World Health Organization (WHO) "Analgesic Ladder" is frequently used as a point of reference. Combinations of drugs are often more effective than one alone:

- **Step 1**: Mild to moderate pain is treated with a non-opioid such as aspirin, acetaminophen, and NSAIDs.
- **Step 2**: Moderate to severe pain unrelieved by Step 1 medications may need opioids, such as codeine, tramadol, or Percocet.
- **Step 3**: Severe pain without relief from Step 1 or Step 2 medications may need stronger opioids, such as morphine, Dilaudid, or MS-Contin.

Note: Meperidine (Demerol) should not be used for long-term pain control because prolonged use may result in dependence, high doses may cause seizures, and a metabolite of meperidine (normeperidine) may accumulate. It is short acting and peaks quickly. It may be indicated for occasional use for the treatment of acute pain, such as that associated with dressing changes.

Pain Medication for Different Types of Wound Pain

Pain medication should be given on a regular schedule, not PRN, for pain that is cyclic or persistent. It should be given 30 minutes prior to painful treatments or dressing changes and again afterwards for non-cyclic pain. The patient should rate the pain before and after pain medication, and dosages should be increased until relief is obtained, or another analgesic should be tried or added to the pain medication regime. Pain medication should be given on schedule even if the patient can sleep, since this does preclude severe pain.

- **Nociceptive pain**, both somatic and visceral, responds to non-opioids, such as acetaminophen or the NSAIDs, and opioid medications, such as acetaminophen with codeine, hydrocodone with acetaminophen or ibuprofen, propoxyphene, morphine, fentanyl, or oxycodone.
- **Neuropathic pain** can be relieved with the adjuvants, such as the tricyclic antidepressants amitriptyline, nortriptyline, or desipramine. Anticonvulsants such as gabapentin or pregabalin are also helpful. Topical and local anesthetics may also be administered. Anesthesia may be indicated for treatments causing severe pain.

Non-Analgesic Pain Control Measures

Non-analgesic pain control measures begin with good communication between the patient and the healthcare provider and an assessment of the causes of pain, which can then be targeted for pain reduction.

- **Cleansing of wound**: Use normal saline and gentle flushing of wound rather than cytotoxic agents, such as antiseptics, which may cause burning and discomfort.
- **Peri-wound care**: Use skin sealants to protect intact skin from maceration and skin barriers over denuded skin.
- **Wound debridement**: Use autolysis when possible.
- **Dressings**: Select dressings with the goal of reducing pain as well as healing the wound. Moisture-retentive dressings often decrease pain. Avoid wet-to-dry dressings. Decrease frequency of dressing changes if possible.
- **Inflammation**: Elevate limb if indicated and provide medications to control inflammation.
- **Edema**: Elevate limbs and use compression dressings and sequential compression pumps as indicated.
- **Positioning**: Use body supports to stabilize wounds when possible, use turning sheets, and try splinting or immobilizing a wound area.

Infection Control

Minimizing Risk of Infection

Wound Care Measures

Procedures for wound care should prevent infection of the wound and should prevent the spread of infection to others. A clean "no-touch" method for dressing changes and wound care is currently recommended. Clean gloves (rather than sterile) are used, but dressings, gauze, swabs, or solutions that directly contact the open area of the wound should be sterile. Any container, such as a syringe or squeeze bottle, used to irrigate the wound should be sterile as well. Wounds should be kept clean and debrided. Antimicrobials should be used as indicated and wound cultures done. Standard precautions should be used with handwashing both before and after treatment of a wound, even with glove use, and before contact with other parts of the body. If any wound irrigation is done that involves fluid under pressure, staff should wear personal protective equipment (gloves, gown, mask, and eye shield) to protect them and other patients from contamination with infective material.

Cleansing Procedures and Solutions

Cleansing methods should remove surface bacteria, but cleansing must be done carefully to prevent damage to tissue. Wounds should be cleansed at each dressing change. Exudate may be removed carefully with soft gauze or swabs by wiping from the center outward, using a new piece of gauze or swab for each wipe. The wound should then be irrigated to mechanically remove exudate or debris. Irrigation under pressure has been found to cleanse wounds effectively while reducing trauma and infection.

- Optimum pressure is 8-12 psi
- <4 psi is inadequate
- >15 psi can cause trauma or force bacteria into tissue

Low-pressure irrigation with a 250 mL squeeze bottle delivers 4.5 psi while a 60 mL piston irrigation syringe delivers 4.2 psi. High-pressure irrigation (8-12 psi) utilizing a 35-cc syringe with an 18- to 19-gauge angiocath provides good cleansing. Irrigation solution should be sterile normal saline instead of antimicrobial/antibacterial solutions, which are cytotoxic and may delay healing.

Sterile and Clean Techniques for Wound Care

Sterile technique is most commonly used in acute care facilities for procedures that are invasive and pose the risk of infection or that involve sharp debridement of tissue. It is important for those who are immunocompromised, chronically ill (e.g., diabetic), elderly, or children. A sterile field is prepared and sterile equipment and dressings are used, with care to maintain principles of sterility.

Clean technique can save money in supplies and time and will not increase the rate of infected wounds when done properly. It is most commonly used in the home environment, physician's offices, and long-term care facilities for dressing changes that do not involve debridement and with patients who are not considered high risk. A clean field is prepared and clean gloves used. If equipment, such as forceps, is used, it must be sterile, but the usual sterile-only-touches-sterile rules do not apply. Dressings may be clean or sterile.

Principles of Sterility

Principles of sterility help to determine what things and areas are sterile and what types of activities constitute contamination:

1. Sterile only touches sterile.
2. Sterile objects should not be wet (poly-lined fields may be wet with sterile fluids only).
3. The outer wrapping of sterile packages is considered contaminated.
4. There should be a one-inch border between sterile and non-sterile area.
5. Sterile drapes hanging over the side of the table are considered unsterile.
6. One should always face the sterile field.
7. Sterile fields must be above the waist as anything below the waist is considered contaminated.
8. All sterile items, including gloved hands, must be held in front of the person and above the waist.
9. Avoid reaching or passing supplies over the sterile field.
10. When pouring sterile solutions onto a container on the sterile field, the bottle should not touch the container and should not splash.
11. Coughing or talking over a sterile field can contaminate the field.

Sterile Field

Two persons can prepare a sterile field. A sterile drape is first placed upon a surface that has been disinfected and dried. The drape is handled only by the edges and is placed upon the surface without touching the surface with the sterile gloves. Any overhang is considered not sterile. One person assists by using clean hands to open packages. The other person scrubs the hands and dons sterile gloves. The assistant opens packages so that the sterile provider may reach in to get the contents without contaminating them. The contents are then placed on the sterile field away from the edges. Items that are not sterile, such as medication vials, are held by the assistant so that the sterile provider may insert a needle without touching the vial to evacuate the contents. One person can prepare the field by placing a sterile drape on the surface and by opening packages and carefully dumping the contents on the drape, rearranging them later while wearing sterile gloves.

Adequate Disinfection of Equipment Used in Wound Treatments

Most cases of nosocomial infections caused by equipment are a result of failure to follow **disinfection guidelines** established by the manufacturer or the facility. Studies have shown that up to 87% of healthcare equipment that was tested had contamination by bacteria. The nature of a device guides the disinfection and cleaning. Devices that are used during invasive procedures require the highest level of disinfection and sterilization. Equipment must first be cleansed of gross contaminants using chemical and mechanical means, then disinfected and sterilized as required by guidelines. Equipment that includes moisture is especially prone to harboring harmful microorganisms. Channels that contain moisture must be rinsed and dried with 70% alcohol solution and forced air. If a patient wound is infected, one must use equipment that can be dedicated to that patient or is disposable if possible.

STANDARDS AND PRECAUTIONS FOR PERSONAL PROTECTIVE EQUIPMENT

The CDC provides standards for the use of protective equipment, based on diagnosis and condition:

- **Standard precautions** (for all patients) include protection from all blood and body fluids and include the use of gloves, face barriers, and gowns as needed to avoid being splashed with fluids.
- **Airborne precautions** require respiratory precautions (a mask) to be worn if the patient has suspected or confirmed tuberculosis.
- **Droplet precautions** (measles, influenza, etc.) require staff and visitors who are within 3 feet of the patient to wear masks.
- **Contact precautions** (for those with infections, such as *Staphylococcus aureus)* include using gloves as for standard precautions, but they should immediately be removed and hands sanitized after contact with infective material. A clean protective gown should be worn inside the room for close contact with the patient and any type of patient care.

HAND HYGIENE STANDARD PRECAUTIONS

According to hand hygiene standard precautions, hands should be washed with soap and water for at least 15 seconds to remove visible soiling whenever exposed to patient-related surfaces, directly before patient contact, and before and after wearing gloves. When hands do not have visible soiling, they may be disinfected with the use of an alcohol-based hand rub. These rubs are more effective than soap and water when all surfaces of the hands are in contact with the rub. If there is a chance of spore contamination, the hands should be washed with antimicrobial soap and water. Healthcare workers in contact with patients who are at high risk for infection should not wear jewelry, artificial fingernails, or extenders. When dressing or treating a wound, hands should be washed before touching other portions of the patient or anything in the room. Surgical scrubbing should include using antimicrobial soap and the scrubbing of the hands and forearms for at least 2 to 6 minutes. This should be followed by an alcohol-based scrub and drying before donning sterile gloves.

CONTACT PRECAUTIONS

Contact precautions are used for patients with infected wounds that may contaminate the environment because of the virulent nature of the microorganism, uncontained drainage, or inability to cooperate on the part of the patient. The patient is placed in a private room or with patients with the same microorganism if possible. Gloves should be worn whenever entering the room and gloves removed and hands washed when exiting the room. A gown must be worn whenever there is a chance of touching the patient or surfaces in the room and always if there is uncontained wound drainage. The patient should only leave the room if it is unavoidable. If transporting, one must ensure wounds are well covered. Equipment should be dedicated to the patient and not shared. The room, furnishings and equipment must be cleaned and disinfected as needed and when the patient is discharged according to facility policy. Waste is double-bagged and handled as hazardous waste according to policy.

Exam Room Preparation and Cleaning

Equipment and Supply Set Up for Basic Wound Care Procedures

All necessary equipment and supplies should be gathered and ready for use before carrying out a wound care procedure, and the patient should be positioned so that the wound is clearly visible and easily accessible by the healthcare provider. The **equipment and supply set up** for basic wound care procedures may vary depending upon the type of wound, but generally includes:

- Adequate lighting (overhead, lamp)
- Hazardous waste container in which to place contaminated dressings and supplies
- Bedside stand or table on which to place supplies
- Irrigating set up with NS to cleanse the wound
- Antiseptic to apply about the wound perimeter
- Both sterile and non-sterile gloves as well as appropriate PPE
- Water-resistant under pads to place under the site of the wound, especially important if irrigating the wound
- Dressing supplies, including sterile dressings, cleansing swabs, and sterile field with sterile forceps (if needed)
- Any medications that may be utilized, such as lidocaine or enzymes

Cleaning of the Patient Environment

The facility policies for the cleaning of patient care areas must follow CDC guidelines for preventing the transmission of infectious agents in healthcare settings. This affects patients with uncontained wound drainage or wound infections. These patients should be in a separate room whenever possible, depending on the microorganism involved. Equipment and furnishings in the room should be cleaned of soil on a daily basis and as needed with an EPA-registered disinfectant. This includes all surfaces touched by the patient, including beds, bedrails, over-bed tables, bedside tables, phone, call bell, TV controls, and bathroom surfaces. Cleaning equipment should be dedicated to use in that room if possible. Terminal disinfection procedures should be followed when the patient is discharged.

Cleaning of Rooms Between Patients

Patients with wounds are at high risk of developing infections with multidrug-resistant organisms and developing infections from environmental transmission (especially if patients have wounds that are draining) because they are often diabetic, paralyzed, and/or debilitated. **Treatment rooms** should be thoroughly cleaned and disinfected between patients, including not only horizontal surfaces but also high-touch surfaces, such as doorknobs, TV controls, call lights, handles, and faucets. If blood or body fluids are evident, these should be removed with wet soapy water prior to disinfection. Reusable equipment used with the patient during treatment, such as blood pressure cuffs, should be cleaned and disinfected. When possible, disposable equipment or individualized equipment should be used to decrease chances of cross contamination. Healthcare providers should utilize standard precautions, including face shields if splashing may occur and should wear appropriate gowns and gloves to avoid contamination of their clothing. Wound care supply carts should be left outside of the treatment room.

Cleaning a Whirlpool Tank

The American Physical Therapy Association (APTA) guide for whirlpool cleansing should be followed:

1. Full personal protective gear should be worn by the person doing the cleaning.
2. Detergent is first used to scrub the inside of tanks, pipes, drains, thermometers, and turbines and all are rinsed.
3. The tank is then filled with hot water with a disinfectant and left for at least 10 minutes, after which it is drained and rinsed.
4. The agitator is immersed in a separate container with disinfectant and hot water and allowed to run for 10 minutes.
5. All equipment is dried with clean towels and then covered.

Hydrotherapy equipment, Hoyer lifts, and transfer equipment must also be cleansed after use. All other equipment and surfaces in the room should be wiped with a germicidal solution due to possible aerosol contamination during the whirlpool.

Levels of Cleaning and Disinfection

The levels of cleaning and disinfection include:

1. **Decontamination**: Makes equipment safe to handle while cleaning, uses 0.5% chlorine solution to decrease microorganisms.
2. **Cleaning**: The removal of gross contamination by using soap and water and scrubbing.
3. **Low-level disinfection**: The removal of SOME microorganisms by using disinfectant.
4. **Intermediate-level disinfection**: The removal of MOST microorganisms by using disinfectant.
5. **High-level disinfection**: The removal of ALL microorganisms (except spores) by using disinfectants, steam, or boiling.
6. **Sterilization**: The removal of ALL microorganisms by using high-pressure steam autoclave, dry heat, radiation, or chemical sterilants.
7. **Reprocessing**: The process that consists of cleaning, high-level disinfection, and drying.

Care Planning

Psychosocial Issues

Effects of Wounds on Patient's Psychological Response

The cause of a wound may affect the patient's and the family's psychological response:

- Traumatic wounds can serve to remind the person of the event involved with its occurrence. Each dressing change, pain, and disability from a wound reminds the person of this disruption in his or her life. Some patients may cope by refusing to see the wound or to be involved in its care until they have progressed to a more accepting phase in their adjustment. Some may react by demanding attention to the wound by others even if the wound is progressing.
- Cancer wounds may cause fear, anxiety, and depression, reminding the person of the disease.
- Wounds sustained through the fault of the patient or from carelessness may be embarrassing or shame producing. Family members may blame the patient.
- Patients coping with a disease or disability, such as quadriplegia, may not have the emotional energy to cope with the reality of a wound as well and may be overwhelmed.

Psychological Support Needed by Patients and Families When Diagnosed with a Wound

Both the patients and families are in need of psychological support when a patient is diagnosed with a wound. The care provider must recognize that after diagnosis, patients and families may go through stages of anger, denial, fear, and frustration and may be psychologically unable to cope with caring for a wound. Patients need positive support and understanding during this period, helping them to reach acceptance and encouraging them to participate in wound care one step at a time. Patients and their families may have many concerns that they are afraid to address, so the care provider must openly address common concerns, especially fear of pain, disability, and disfigurement. Patients who have a plan for pain control and have realistic explanations about disability feel less threatened. Disfigurement must be discussed, and a plan for treatment that minimizes negative results must be developed. Reassurance that the wound will heal encourages hope and positive expectations that the entire ordeal will end at some point in the future.

Social Isolation Due to Wounds

Physical mobility may be affected by the wound and by pain, contributing to social isolation by keeping a patient close to home. The need to rest or elevate the wound cuts down on ambulation. Treatments or dressing changes can take much time out of the day. If patients must travel to a clinic or office to have these treatments, then this takes time from their normal schedule and responsibilities. Patients may experience fatigue from poor sleep and side effects from medications such as antibiotics or pain medication, making them less likely to seek social contact. The fear of further injury to the wound can restrict the person's activities and the places that they are willing to go. The appearance of the wound, dressings, or the type of clothes or shoes that are necessary may also limit the person's desire to go out in public.

Psychosocial Issues Caused by Wounds with Odor and Drainage

Wounds with odor and excessive exudate may have a profound psychological impact on the patient, who often feels embarrassed and ashamed. Some may try to mask the odor with cologne or perfumes, but this often compounds the problem. The patient may become depressed and avoid social interaction, becoming increasingly isolated. Family and friends may indicate that they find the odor or drainage offensive. The patient often feels a loss of self-esteem. Intimacy is often avoided by the patient or his or her partner, making the person feel unwanted. Cancerous wounds may serve as a constant reminder of impending death. With heavily draining wounds, the need for bulky dressings impacts the type of clothing the patient can wear, making the person feel unattractive. Patients need reassurance that the odor or drainage can be contained and need instruction in methods to manage the wound, such as cleansing the wound properly, using charcoal or special wound deodorants, and applying dressings that contain the drainage between changes.

Psychological Effects of Acute or Traumatic Wounds

An acute or sudden traumatic wound suddenly puts a person who is healthy into the role of a patient. The wound gets all of the patient and family's attention. The patient's role and responsibilities are impacted and changed by the presence of the wound. The traumatic wound may cause emotions that were previously hidden to emerge, stressing the patient's coping mechanisms and causing emotional crisis. It is not until the wound heals that the patient resumes being the "normal" individual that he or she was prior to the wound. The care provider can help the patient to learn coping mechanisms and ways to resume normalcy prior to complete healing to ease the feeling of being a different person due to the presence of the wound.

Psychological Effects of Chronic Wounds

A wound that is present for years can cause a loss of hope, depression, and lack of compliance by the patient who has no reward when the wound fails to heal. Activities are focused around the wound and planned around any pain or disability caused by the wound, such as difficulty walking. Sleep can be altered and lack of energy can hamper ADLs over time. Patients may go through the grieving process. Each dressing change is accompanied by relief if it is improved or depression if it is not.

- Patients may choose to live with the wound and continue with normal life activities, modified to accommodate the wound.
- Others may stay in and wait for wound healing to occur to resume life as before.
- Patients may find comfort from comparing themselves to others with wounds or chronic illnesses.
- Some may feel well except for the wound, and be able to continue life while coping with the healing process.
- Some may accept the wound as a part of life and growing old.

Impact of Wounds on Females vs. Males

Gender issues related to wounds are a matter of ongoing research. Studies have shown that males with wounds tend to report more of an impact from pain and limitations in mobility than females. They also lose more sleep when a wound is present and tend to be socially isolated by a wound. They may feel emotionally challenged more than females who have wounds. Females feel less energetic and less able to cope physically. They are also affected socially when a wound is present. However, studies of diabetic ulcers indicate that female gender along with small ulcer size and lack of infection was predictive of better healing. Additionally, females tend to have lower incidence of ulcers, possibly because of smaller size resulting in less pressure on the foot and less severe neuropathy.

Effects of Age on Psychological Reaction to Wounds

Studies have indicated that younger patients tend to be more negatively impacted by wounds than older people, who may have more effective coping abilities and can more easily adapt to physical restrictions. Younger people are more active and social, and any activity restriction causes more of a change in their lifestyle. Young patients may not have had as many previous experiences in coping with illness or disability as older patients, and their expectations are often different. The support network for young patients may be narrower than for older, who may, for example, have children to assist them. Younger people often have less job and financial security, which increases stress. However, the group is not always an accurate representation of the individual. Some young people cope well while some older people react negatively to wounds.

Helping Patients with Disfiguring Wounds

Disfiguring wounds take a daily emotional toll on the patient. Family reactions to the wound can adjust over time, but social encounters can result in stares and reactions of pity, disgust, repulsion, and disdain from others, causing a loss of self-esteem and negative feelings about the wound. Some disfiguring wounds, such as post-mastectomy, may impact a person's sexuality and self-identity. The care provider can provide acceptance, treat the wound in a matter-of-fact way without negative reactions, and suggest practical ways to camouflage or minimize the appearance of the wound. The care provider can discuss reconstructive options and differences that will occur with healing such as less discoloration and swelling, provide encouragement and positivity about the healing process, and inquire about the patient's general well-being and any other problems the patient may have. This emphasizes that the patient is a person with a wound, not a wound alone.

Impact of a Wound on Family Caregivers

The burden of caring for a loved one with a wound is stressful. Much time is spent on wound care and helping the patient with ADLs. Other family members may feel slighted or burdened with more chores and responsibility. **Caregivers** are conflicted by feelings of wanting to help the patient and yet resenting the need to spend so much time doing so. They may react with anger or even abuse. A lengthy healing period stresses coping and the caregiver may need to have help at times to allow time away from the patient or to take care of other matters. The patient may feel helpless and a burden or may be demanding and depend on the caregiver for emotional and physical support. Caregivers who are older or have their own health problems can be stretched to the limit. Providers can offer the caregiver an outlet for emotions and concerns and help them to find ways to meet their own needs as well as the patient's during this trying time.

Financial Impact of Wounds and Ulcers

The wound or ulcer may make it difficult for people to continue their jobs due to pain or the need to rest the limb. This can affect compliance with the healing regime. Patients without savings, another wage earner in the family, or other resources may have to tap into equity in their homes or take out loans to meet **financial obligations**. Patients may lose their jobs or be forced to quit or take early retirement. Even with health insurance, patients may have out-of-pocket expenses, such as for dressings, medications, the cost of transportation for treatments, and help for ADLs or housekeeping. Patients may be eligible for public assistance, but this may cause them shame and provide less income than they need. The care provider should assess financial status and make referrals as needed to local agencies that can help the patient. The choice of dressings and treatments needs to be made with the best option meeting the need for optimal healing combined with the need to contain costs for patients.

Impacts of Healthcare Professionals on Patients' Perception

Healthcare professionals affect the patient's psychological reactions by their words, expressions, and actions concerning the wound. A reaction of disappointment, surprise, disgust, or disdain causes the patient to feel shame, embarrassment, imperfection, vulnerability, and other negative feelings. Caregivers also have these reactions. A healthcare professional may assume the patient has the level of knowledge needed to prevent such wounds, implying blame, when in fact the patient does not, but the patient may react with shame and guilt. Healthcare professionals who do not teach the patient about the wound or treatment, give results of tests or measurements, or include the patient in decisions or discussion about the wound can cause the patient to feel negatively towards the person and facility.

Patient-Centered Plan of Care

Identification of Patient Goals and Factors Affecting Care

It is easy to confuse healthcare provider goals with patient goals. Healthcare provider goals involve restoring a patient to the best health possible; however, patients' goals may be very different, or patients may lack defined goals. The only way to help patients to establish goals is to talk to them, helping them arrive at realistic short-term and long-term goals based on their condition and abilities. There are a number of **factors that can affect goals and care**:

- **Functional disability** may prevent a patient from taking the steps needed to reach a goal.
- **Mental status** may be such that a patient is not competent to set goals or to carry out needed actions.
- **Co-morbidity** may result in health problems that interfere with plan of care.
- **Low income** may prevent a patient from buying supplies or getting needed assistance.
- **Social circumstances** may be such that the patient lacks family support or is dependent on others.
- **Smoking** may impact healing.

Preventive, Maintenance, and Curative Goals

Goals should be set with the patient regarding prevention, maintenance, and cure:

- **Preventive goals**: Measures to prevent disease or disability or to prevent deterioration or complications of an existing disorder. May include screening (BP, Pap smear, mammograms, blood glucose), disease education, fall prevention, smoking cessation, substance abuse rehabilitation, vaccinations, nutritional counseling, and exercise.
- **Maintenance goals**: Measures to control an existing disorder in order to maintain status. May include therapy (OT, PT, ST), education, ongoing lifestyle changes, supervision, ongoing assessment, medications, blood glucose management, and treatment. Maintenance therapy may follow primary therapy for some diseases, such as cancer, in order to maintain status.
- **Curative goals**: Measures intended to cure disease rather than simply to alleviate symptoms or pain. May include medications, casting (as for broken limbs), radiotherapy, dialysis, transfusions, chemotherapy, physical therapy, rehabilitation therapy, and surgical interventions. *Note: Curative treatments without the intent to cure are also sometimes used for palliation.*

Access to Care

A number of factors may influence a patient's access to care:

- **Proximity to medical services**: Some geographic areas have more medical services than others. For example, some rural areas lack both hospitals and physicians. Cutting-edge treatments may be unavailable in some areas.
- **Socioeconomic status**: Lack of insurance or money to pay for medical services prevents many people from seeking medical care or complying with treatments. Many cannot afford to pay for prescription drugs or supplies.
- **Language differences**: Non-English speakers may not be able to communicate needs or to understand information, such as the treatment plan.
- **Health literacy**: Some may have little knowledge and understanding of anatomy, physiology, disease, and medical treatments.
- **Disability status**: Disabilities may have a profound effect on access to care or very little, depending on the type of disability and the resources available, but some disabilities impair mobility and the ability to access care.
- **Transportation**: Private and public transportation may be unavailable or cost prohibitive.
- **Race and ethnicity**: Inequalities faced by minority populations often extend to medical services. Some individuals live in poor neighborhoods that provide little access to medical services.

Issues Related to Assessment of Wounds at End-of-Life

While the primary goals of skin care are to prevent and heal wounds, when patients are near the end-of-life there are a number of issues to assess:

- Hospice care
- Advance directives
- Best interests of the patient

Patients under hospice care are to receive palliative rather than curative treatment, but in the case of wound care, sometimes treatments that are essentially curative are appropriate if they reduce pain and discomfort. The Patient Self-Determination Act allows people to refuse treatment when they are competent to make that decision and to make advance directives about end-of-life care, and this must be respected in relation to wound care. As systems deteriorate near the end of life, patients are prone to pressure sores, so deciding what must be treated and what treatment is futile can be difficult. Frequently changing the patient's position to prevent pressure may increase pain and discomfort. These decisions must be individualized.

Palliative Care

Palliative care is not curative (although it may be carried out in conjunction with curative treatments) but aims to provide emotional support and comfort measures, such as relief of pain, nausea, vomiting, dyspnea, and other symptoms. Palliative care is often carried out as part of hospice care but should be a consideration in the care of all patients. Palliative care may include oxygen, positioning, complementary therapies, analgesia, stool softeners, and antiemetics. Palliative wound care focuses on managing and preventing the symptoms associated with wounds, such as wound infections, discharge, and odor, rather than solely on healing the wounds. Skin breakdown is a common finding as patients near death and cutaneous perfusion decreases. Strategies should include measures to reduce risk of further skin and ulcer breakdown through proper positioning and application of appropriate dressings, to manage symptoms that are present, to attend to the emotional needs of the patient and the patient's family, and to provide care to existing wounds.

Therapeutic Relationships

Religious Objections to Treatment

Jehovah's Witnesses

Jehovah's Witnesses have traditionally shunned transfusions and blood products as part of their religious beliefs. In 2004, the *Watchtower,* a Jehovah's Witness publication, presented a guide for members. When medical care indicates the need for blood transfusion or blood products and the patient and/or family members are practicing Jehovah's Witnesses, this may present a conflict. It's important to approach the patient/family with full information and reasons for the transfusion or blood components without being judgmental, allowing them to express their feelings. In fact, studies show that while adults often refuse transfusions for themselves, they frequently allow their children to receive blood products, so one should never assume that an individual would refuse blood products based on the religion alone. Jehovah's Witnesses can receive fractionated blood cells, thus allowing hemoglobin-based blood substitutes. The following guidelines are provided to church members:

Basic **blood standards for Jehovah's Witnesses**:

- **Not acceptable**: Whole blood: red cells, white cells, platelets, plasma.
- **Acceptable**: Fractions from red cells, white cells, platelets, and plasma.

Christian Scientists

Christian Science, a religion developed by Mary Baker Eddy in 1879, promotes the belief that sickness is most effectively treated through prayer alone. While Christian Scientists do not avoid all medical interventions, their beliefs are conservative regarding medical treatment. Most notably, Christian Scientists, for the most part, do not believe in vaccinations and may only agree to such if required by law, as they do acknowledge the importance of community health. They have widely appreciated the use of exemptions from mandatory vaccines, but as these exemptions have become more limited, religious leaders have given their members the right to decide upon vaccinations.

Impact of Culture and Religion on Dietary Preferences

When performing a dietary assessment, the nurse should remember that culture and religion might dictate which foods and spices are used. The manner in which food is prepared, cooked, and served may also be specified. The utensils used at the meal as well as the persons who may eat together may be important. Mealtimes and required fasts should be determined. Holidays may be accompanied by particular foods. Alcohol (including extracts made with alcohol) and caffeine may be prohibited. The culture may also consider obesity a sign of affluence and success. The nurse should evaluate the foods that are eaten in light of the patient's medical condition. The patient may not wish to eat the usual hospital fare and may need to have a special diet prepared or food brought from home. The nurse can guide the patient and family to foods that are acceptable and within the patient's requirements for health.

Therapeutic Communication

Facilitating Communication

Therapeutic communication begins with respect for the patient/family and the assumption that all communication, verbal and nonverbal, has meaning. Listening must be done empathetically. The following are some techniques that facilitate communication.

Introduction:

- Make a personal introduction and use the patient's name: "Mrs. Brown, I am Susan Williams, your nurse."

Encouragement:

- Use an open-ended opening statement: "Is there anything you'd like to discuss?"
- Acknowledge comments: "Yes," and "I understand."
- Allow silence and observe nonverbal behavior rather than trying to force conversation. Ask for clarification if statements are unclear.
- Reflect statements back (use sparingly): Patient: "I hate this hospital." Nurse: "You hate this hospital?"

Empathy:

- Make observations: "You are shaking," and "You seem worried."
- Recognize feelings:
  - Patient: "I want to go home."
  - Nurse: "It must be hard to be away from your home and family."
- Provide information as honestly and completely as possible about condition, treatment, and procedures and respond to the patient's questions and concerns.

Exploration:

- Verbally express implied messages:
  - Patient: "This treatment is too much trouble."
  - Nurse: "You think the treatment isn't helping you?"
- Explore a topic but allow the patient to terminate the discussion without further probing: "I'd like to hear how you feel about that."

Orientation:

- Indicate reality:
  - Patient: "Someone is screaming."
  - Nurse: "That sound was an ambulance siren."
- Comment on distortions without directly agreeing or disagreeing:
  - Patient: "That nurse promised I didn't have to walk again."
  - Nurse: "Really? That's surprising because the doctor ordered physical therapy twice a day."

Collaboration:

- Work together to achieve better results: "Maybe if we talk about this, we can figure out a way to make the treatment easier for you."

Validation:

- Seek validation: "Do you feel better now?" or "Did the medication help you breathe better?"

Avoiding Non-Therapeutic Communication

While using therapeutic communication is important, it is equally important to avoid interjecting **non-therapeutic communication**, which can block effective communication. *Avoid the following:*

- Meaningless clichés: "Don't worry. Everything will be fine." "Isn't it a nice day?"
- Providing advice: "You should..." or "The best thing to do is...." It's better when patients ask for advice to provide facts and encourage the patient to reach a decision.
- Inappropriate approval that prevents the patient from expressing true feeling or concerns:
  - Patient: "I shouldn't cry about this."
  - Nurse: "That's right! You're an adult!"
- Asking for an explanation of behavior that is not directly related to patient care and requires analysis and explanation of feelings: "Why are you so upset?"
- Agreeing with rather than accepting and responding to patient's statements can make it difficult for the patient to change his or her statement or opinion later: "I agree with you," or "You are right."
- Making negative judgments: "You should stop arguing with the nurses."
- Devaluing the patient's feelings: "Everyone gets upset at times."
- Disagreeing directly: "That can't be true," or "I think you are wrong."
- Defending against criticism: "The doctor is not being rude; he's just very busy today."
- Changing the subject to avoid dealing with uncomfortable topics;
  - Patient: "I'm never going to get well."
  - Nurse: "Your family will be here in just a few minutes."
- Making inappropriate literal responses, even as a joke, especially if the patient is at all confused or having difficulty expressing ideas:
  - Patient: "There are bugs crawling under my skin."
  - Nurse: "I'll get some bug spray,"
- Challenging the patient to establish reality often just increases confusion and frustration:
  - "If you were dying, you wouldn't be able to yell and kick!"

Communicating with Patients with Disabilities

Guidelines for communicating with individuals with disabilities:

- Do not assume that the person with disabilities also has impaired cognition.
- Always treat the person with respect and dignity.
- Use first names with the patient if asked to do so, but start out formally as with any patient.
- Offer to shake hands even when a prosthesis is present.
- Be patient if communication is impaired.
- Offer assistance, but allow the patient to tell you what is helpful; otherwise don't assist.
- When a wheelchair is used, sit down so the patient does not have to strain their neck to speak with you.
- If providing directions, consider the obstacles that may be in the way and assist the person to find an appropriate way around them.

Communication with Patients with Cognitive Disabilities

The person with cognitive disabilities may be easily distracted, so verbal communication should be attempted in a quiet area:

- Address people with dignity and respect.
- Do not try to discuss abstract ideas but stick with concrete topics.
- Keep words and sentences very simple and try rephrasing when necessary. People may have difficulty in distinguishing your spoken words and deriving the meaning from them.
- Be very patient with people's attempts to speak to you since they may have difficulty in processing thoughts and changing them into spoken words.
- Use objects around you and gestures to illustrate your words since the patient may also use pointing and gesturing when unable to find the words to communicate with you. The person may prefer written communication, although some may be unable to read.
- Use touch to convey your regard during communication, as this is recognized by the patient as reassurance of your care and concern for them.
- Give a few instructions at a time as to not overwhelm them.

Communicating with Deaf or Hearing-Impaired Patients

Communicating with a person with deafness or hearing impairment:

- Try to communicate in a quiet environment if possible.
- Wave or touch the person to let him or her know you are trying to communicate.
- Determine the method the person uses to communicate: sign language, lip reading, hearing devices, or writing.
- Fingerspell or use some signs if able to do so.
- Address the person directly when you speak even though the person may be looking at an interpreter or your lips.
- Look at the person as the interpreter tells you what was said.
- Speak slowly so the interpreter can keep up with you.
- If the person reads lips, face the person and speak clearly and normally, using normal volume.
- If writing a communication, do not speak while writing.
- Do not be afraid to check that the person understands you, and ask questions if you do not understand the person.

Communication with People with Low Vision or Blindness

Communicating with a person with low vision or blindness:

- Greet the person with low vision or blindness, identifying yourself and others present.
- Always say goodbye when you are leaving.
- Alert the person to written communications, such as warning signs or printed notices.
- Face the person and touch briefly on the arm to let the person know you are speaking to him or her if you are in a group.
- Speak at normal loudness.
- Make any directions given specific in terms of the length of walk and obstacles, such as stairs.
- Use the position of hands on a clock face to give directions (potatoes at 3 o'clock) as well as using *right* or *left*.
- Mention sounds that the person may hear in transit or on arrival at a destination.

Communicating with a Patient on a Ventilator

When a patient on a ventilator is conscious, he or she may still be able to communicate by blinking, nodding, shaking the head, or pointing to a picture or word board:

- If the person is able to write, try to reposition the IV line to leave the dominant hand free to communicate.
- Discuss the need for communication with the physician and ask if a valve or an electric larynx can be used to permit speech.
- Help the patient practice lip reading of single words.
- Remember the patient's glasses or hearing aids when attempting to communicate.
- Enlist the aid of a speech therapist if there is frustration on the part of the patient and family due to communication difficulty.

Communicating with Persons with Speech Problems Due to a Stroke

Methods to communicate with stroke patients with speech problems:

- **Dysarthria**: Patients have problems forming the words to speak them aloud. Give them time to communicate, offer them a picture board or other means of communicating, and give encouragement to family members who are frustrated with the difficulty of trying to communicate.
- **Expressive aphasia**: The patients' efforts at speech come out garbled when they try to say sentences, but single words may be clear. Encourage the patients to try to write and to practice the sounds of the alphabet. Resist the urge to finish sentences for the patients.
- **Receptive aphasia**: The patients have a problem comprehending the speech they hear. Communicate in simple terms and speak slowly. Test comprehension of the written word as an alternative method of communication.
- **Global aphasia**: The patient has both receptive and expressive aphasia. Use simple, clear, slow speech augmented by pictures and gestures.

COMMUNICATION PROBLEMS OF PATIENTS WITH PARKINSON'S DISEASE

Parkinson's disease causes problems with speaking in the majority (75–90%) of patients. The reason for this is not clear but may relate to increasing rigidity and changes in movement. Speech is often very low-pitched or hoarse, given in a monotone and with a soft voice. Speech production may decrease because of the effort required to speak. **Speech therapy** can develop exercises for the patient that can assist them in remembering to speak slowly and carefully, as patients are not always aware that their **communication** is impaired:

- Allow time for the patient to communicate, asking for repetition if you do not understand the message.
- Help family by teaching ways to facilitate communication with the patient and encouraging them to assist the patient to do the exercises provided by the therapist.
- If speech volume is very low, suggest amplification devices that can be obtained through speech therapy.

COMMUNICATION WITH PATIENTS WITH PSYCHIATRIC PROBLEMS

Persons with psychiatric disorders appreciate being addressed with respect, dignity, and honesty:

- Speak simply and clearly, repeating as necessary.
- Encourage patients to discuss their concerns regarding treatment and medications to improve compliance.
- Use good eye contact and be attentive to your body language messages.
- Be alert, but unless the person is known to be violent, try to relax and listen to them.
- Don't try to avoid words or phrases pertaining to psychiatric problems, but if you do say something inappropriate, apologize honestly to the patient.
- Offer patients outlets for their thoughts and feelings.
- Learn more about their disorder and ways to use therapeutic communication to help them with their problem, such as re-orienting them as needed.

CULTURAL COMPETENCE

Different cultures view health and illness from very different perspectives, and patients often come from a mix of many cultures, so the nurse must be not only accepting of cultural differences but must be sensitive and aware. There are a number of characteristics that are important for a nurse to have **cultural competence**:

- **Appreciating diversity**: This must be grounded in information about other cultures and understanding of their value systems.
- **Assessing own cultural perspectives**: Self-awareness is essential to understanding potential biases.
- **Understanding intercultural dynamics**: This must include understanding ways in which cultures cooperate, differ, communicate, and reach understanding.
- **Recognizing institutional culture**: Each institutional unit (hospital, clinic, office) has an inherent set of values that may be unwritten but is accepted by the staff.
- **Adapting patient service to diversity**: This is the culmination of cultural competence as it is the point of contact between cultures.

CULTURAL CHARACTERISTICS

HISPANIC PATIENTS

Many areas of the country have large populations of Hispanics and Hispanic Americans. As always, it's important to recognize that cultural generalizations don't always apply to individuals. Recent immigrants, especially, have cultural needs that the nurse must understand:

- Many Hispanics are Catholic and may like the nurse to make arrangements for a priest to visit.
- Large extended families may come to visit to support the patient and family, so patients should receive clear explanations about how many visitors are allowed, but some flexibility may be required.

- Language barriers may exist as some may have limited or no English skills, so translation services should be available around the clock.
- Hispanic culture encourages outward expressions of emotions, so family may react strongly to news about a patient's condition, and people who are ill may expect some degree of pampering, so extra attention to the patient/family members may alleviate some of their anxiety.

Caring for Hispanic and Hispanic American patients requires understanding of cultural differences:

- Some immigrant Hispanics have very little formal education, so medical information may seem very complex and confusing, and they may not understand the implications or need for follow-up care.
- Hispanic culture perceives time with more flexibility than American culture, so if parents need to be present at a particular time, the nurse should specify the exact time (1:30 PM) and explain the reason rather than saying something more vague, such as "after lunch."
- People may appear to be unassertive or unable to make decisions when they are simply showing respect to the nurse by being deferent.
- In traditional families, the males make decisions, so a woman waits for the father or other males in the family to make decisions about treatment or care.
- Families may choose to use folk medicines instead of Western medical care or may combine the two.
- Children and young women are often sheltered and are taught to be respectful to adults, so they may not express their needs openly.

Middle Eastern Patients

There are considerable cultural differences among Middle Easterners, but religious beliefs about the segregation of males and females are common. It's important to remember that segregating the female is meant to protect her virtue. Female nurses have low status in many countries because they violate this segregation by touching male bodies, so parents may not trust or show respect for the nurse who is caring for their family member. Additionally, male patients may not want to be cared for by female nurses or doctors, and families may be very upset at a female being cared for by a male nurse or physician. When possible, these cultural traditions should be accommodated:

- In Middle Eastern countries, males make decisions, so issues for discussion or decision should be directed to males, such as the father or spouse, and males may be direct in stating what they want, sometimes appearing demanding.
- If a male nurse must care for a female patient, then the family should be advised that *personal care* (such as bathing) will be done by a female while the medical treatments will be done by the male nurse.

Caring for Middle Eastern patients requires understanding of cultural differences:

- Families may practice strict dietary restrictions, such as avoiding pork and requiring that animals be killed in a ritual manner, so vegetarian or kosher meals may be required.
- People may have language difficulties requiring a translator, and same-sex translators should be used if at all possible.
- Families may be accompanied by large extended families that want to be kept informed and whom patients consult before decisions are made.
- Most medical care is provided by female relatives, so educating the family about patient care should be directed at females (with female translators if necessary).
- Outward expressions of grief are considered as showing respect for the dead.
- Middle Eastern families often offer gifts to caregivers. Small gifts (candy) that can be shared should be accepted graciously, but for other gifts, the families should be advised graciously that accepting gifts is against hospital policy.
- Middle Easterners often require less personal space and may stand very close.

Asian Patients

There are considerable differences among different Asian populations, so cultural generalizations may not apply to all, but nurses caring for Asian patients should be aware of common cultural attitudes and behaviors:

- Nurses and doctors are viewed with respect, so traditional Asian families may expect the nurse to remain authoritative and to give directions and may not question, so the nurse should ensure that they understand by having them review material or give demonstrations and should provide explanations clearly, anticipating questions that the family might have but may not articulate.
- Disagreeing is considered impolite. "Yes" may only mean that the person is heard, not that they agree with the person. When asked if they understand, they may indicate that they do even when they clearly do not so as not to offend the nurse.
- Asians may avoid eye contact as an indication of respect. This is especially true of children in relation to adults and of younger adults in relation to elders.

Caring for Asian patients requires understanding of cultural differences:

- Patients/families may not show outward expressions of feelings/grief, sometimes appearing passive. They also avoid public displays of affection. This does not mean that they don't feel, just that they don't show their feelings.
- Families often hide illness and disabilities from others and may feel ashamed about illness.
- Terminal illness is often hidden from the patient, so families may not want patients to know they are dying or seriously ill.
- Families may use cupping, pinching, or applying pressure to injured areas, and this can leave bruises that may appear as abuse, so when bruises are found, the family should be questioned about alternative therapy before assumptions are made.
- Patients may be treated with traditional herbs.
- Families may need translators because of poor or no English skills.
- In traditional Asian families, males are authoritative and make the decisions.

Education and Referral

Patient Education

Education Regarding Risk Factors and Prevention Strategies

Teaching patients and caregivers about risk factors and prevention strategies is an important part of wound management:

- **Limited mobility**: Referral for physical or occupational therapy may be indicated. If patients are unable to change position, caregivers must be taught proper skin care and positioning.
- **Diabetes**: Proper glucose monitoring and control is critical. Patients should avoid going barefoot and should inspect feet daily.
- **Impaired circulation**: Exercises may be indicated. Proper positioning to increase circulation should be stressed. Restrictive socks or clothing should be avoided.
- **Cognitive impairment**: Caregiver should be advised of all necessary treatments and may need to institute safety measures and assist patient with hygiene.
- **Malnutrition**: Diet should be planned and explained, and supplements should be provided. Meals-on-wheels or assistance for food preparation and eating may be necessary.
- **Fecal and urinary contamination**: Medical and dietary instructions should be given to control incontinence, including scheduled voiding. Skin barriers may be needed as well as assistance with hygiene and adult briefs.

Risk of Skin Breakdown

Patient teaching points regarding the risk of skin breakdown include:

- Advise that skin over the tailbone, hips, shoulder blades, heels, inner and outer ankles, inner and outer knees, elbows, and the back of the head should be checked frequently for skin breakdown.
- Teach about the results of pressure on capillaries and the signs of early damage.
- Explain friction and shearing forces.
- Explain the action of urine and feces upon the skin and the need to keep the patient clean and dry.
- Teach techniques needed to move the patient in the bed using a lift sheet or trapeze.
- Stress the need to prevent skin breakdown to avoid lengthy and costly wound care.
- Recommend soaps and lotions, avoiding those that dry skin, based on the general skin condition and the patient's financial resources.
- Advise the patient and caregiver not to hesitate to call the nurse or physician to report any concerns about skin condition.

Education Regarding Lifestyle Changes to Maximize Perfusion

The patient with arterial insufficiency must make lifestyle changes in order to avoid serious complications and/or amputation of the affected limb:

- Maintain adequate hydration to decrease blood viscosity, but avoid caffeine, which is vasoconstrictive.
- Keep pain under control in order to prevent further vasoconstriction.
- Stop smoking, as nicotine has vasoconstrictive properties.
- Begin a graduated walking program to improve tissue oxygenation, decrease pain, and increase activity tolerance.
- Avoid cold and constrictive clothing to avoid vasoconstriction.
- Do careful skin inspection and skin care: drying skin, using emollients and lamb's wool or foam between toes.
- Wear properly fitted, closed-toe shoes and avoid going barefoot.
- Have professional foot and nail care.
- Wear warm socks during cold weather, but avoid hot water bottles, heating pads, or hot bathing temperatures.
- Avoid the use of antiseptics or chemicals except as prescribed.
- Report even small injuries or changes in skin promptly.

Additional Measures to Improve Perfusion

There are a number of additional and more interventional measures which can improve the perfusion to wounds that the patient should be educated on:

- Management of diet and medication to control blood glucose levels, high blood pressure, and lipid levels.
- Aspirin therapy to reduce the danger of clot formation.
- Surgical revascularization to replace damaged vessels.
- Hyperbaric oxygen therapy, which increases available oxygen to tissues by 10-20 times. Blood that is saturated increases perfusion of the tissues. It is indicated for peripheral arterial insufficiency, compromised skin from grafts, and diabetic ulcers.
- Topical hyperbaric oxygen therapy has shown promise in increasing circulation and healing wounds. The topical oxygen increases perfusion to the wound bed itself rather than systemically.
- Circulator Boot therapy, an end-diastolic compression equipment system, is used to treat ulcers of the lower extremity. Compressions coordinate with the end of diastole to increase perfusion. It is FDA approved for the treatment of deficient arterial blood flow.

Management of Nutritional Factors That Affect Wound Healing

Nutritional management must be designed according to individual needs based on many factors, such as age, weight, size, nutritional status, co-morbidity, and size and severity of wound. The average healthy person requires about 0.8 g of protein per kilogram every day (40-70 g). However, if a person has a wound, then not only must the person have adequate calories and general nutrition, but additional daily protein and vitamins as well:

- Protein amounts are increased to 1.25–2.0 g/kg
- Vitamin A 1600–2000 retinal equivalents
- Vitamin C 100–1000 mg
- Zinc 15–30 mg
- B vitamins 200% of RDA
- Iron 20–30 mg

Caloric and fluid intake should be monitored carefully to ensure that the person is eating the food that is served. Gastrointestinal tube feedings or parenteral feedings may be necessary if the person cannot take food and fluids orally. Prealbumin levels should be monitored regularly as well.

Dietary Changes to Add Protein, Calories and Nutrients

There are a number of dietary changes that can add adequate protein, calories, and needed nutrients to the diet. In some people, co-morbid conditions such as diabetes or high cholesterol should be considered because some foods, such as cheese, are high in sodium and fat, which may be restricted.

To **increase protein**:

- Add meat to vegetarian dishes, such as soups and pastas.
- Add milk powder to many foods during preparation.
- Substitute milk for water in soups, hot cereals, and cocoa.
- Add cheese to dishes, such as pastas and casseroles.
- Provide high protein drinks, such as High Protein Ensure.
- Use peanut butter on bread and apples.
- Add extra eggs to dishes, such as custards and meat loaf

To **increase calories**:

- Use whole milk or cream rather than low fat or non-fat milk.
- Add butter, sour cream, or whipping cream to foods.
- Provide frequent snacks.

Nutritional Advice for Patients with Ulcers or Risks for Skin Problems

Diabetic patients and those with ulcers or skin problems should have consultation with a dietitian for an individualized diet that meets healing needs without raising the blood sugar:

- Patients should be advised to drink at least 8 glasses of fluids per day unless there is a contraindication.
- Diets should have increased protein and iron for healing.
- Carbohydrates should be complex, and high-glycemic carbohydrates, which increase blood sugar, should be limited.
- Caloric intake should be determined by the dietitian.
- Eating small meals every few hours is preferable to 3 large meals.
- A dietary supplement may be prescribed up to three times a day to meet nutritional needs.
- Patients and caregivers should have lists of foods that help to provide the nutrients that the patient needs.

Skin Self-Assessment

The areas of the skin that are prone to breakdown should be assessed with the patient and caregiver present and unique findings discussed. This provides a baseline condition for them to reference when they do further assessments of the area:

- Teach how to blanch the skin and how to report signs of redness, abrasion, pallor, changes in skin texture or color, pain, bruising, or swelling.
- Provide pictures and color charts with demonstrations of skin abnormalities to watch for if possible.
- Show how to measure skin lesions or discolorations.
- Stress the importance of communicating areas of concern between caregivers so that changes are noted and monitored and action is taken to prevent breakdown and to bring the concern to the attention of the patient's nurse or physician.

Wound Self-Assessment

The patient must learn to look at the wound and surrounding skin to assess for signs of infection or wound problems. The color of the tissues in the wound, and the amount, color, and odor of exudate should be explained. The patient must be taught to report pain in or around the wound or signs of redness, swelling, warmth, increased exudate or pus, or fever. The condition of the skin around the wound should be noted and reported if there are any signs of maceration or breakdown. The patient should also note whether the wound bed is dry or moist. The patient should be taught how to measure the wound consistently when dressings are changed. The signs of a beefy red healthy wound bed and of the various stages of a healing wound should be illustrated to the patient and caregiver to help them recognize and distinguish a healing wound from a non-healing or infected wound.

Measurement of Wounds

The patient should be taught to measure the wound at the greatest length and width without touching the wound. The patient may also be taught to use two pieces of plastic wrap or a clean plastic bag to trace the wound with a permanent marker. The layers are laid on the wound and the edges are traced onto the top layer. After the ink dries the top layer of the bag is cut off or the top layer of plastic is removed. The patient should label each tracing with the date and time. The bottom layer touching the wound is then disposed of with the old dressing as hazardous waste. One can leave a form for the patient to record the date and measurements so that healing progress can be tracked.

Changing a Dressing at Home

The patient should be alert and able to follow instructions regarding ulcer or wound dressings at home. A caregiver may be present to learn as reinforcement for the patient or to perform dressing changes and care for the patient. Teaching includes:

- Teach the importance of washing hands, using gloves, and disposing of hazardous waste properly.
- Demonstrate the dressing change using clean technique.
- Demonstrate the technique of removing the old dressing slowly to avoid trauma to the wound, then washing and regloving.
- Teach how to assess and measure the wound and the symptoms of infection to be reported. Demonstrate the technique to be used for wound cleansing or irrigation if needed.
- Show how to pad wounds if exudate is present.
- Finally teach the assessment of periwound tissues, how to apply skin protectant if needed, and how to secure the dressing to the site.

Self-Care of Compression Therapy

Teach patients to care for their compression stockings by maintaining two pairs, washing them according to manufacturer's instructions, and replacing them when they lose elasticity in 3 to 6 months. They should inspect skin of the legs and feet daily for breakdown or trauma. Stockings will dry the skin, so they should wash the feet and legs, dry them lightly, and apply a moisturizer without fragrance after removing the stockings for the night. Patients with lymphedema need to understand their disease and the need to control edema continuously. They should be taught skin care and how to apply special treatment when weeping dermatitis is present. Compression garments may be used after decongestive physiotherapy and massage brings edema under control. Exercises to gradually strengthen the calf muscles should be taught to the patient. Patients must comply with compression therapy and exercises to keep lymphedema under control.

Potential Adverse Effects of Compression Therapy

There are a number of potential adverse effects of compression therapy that the patient should monitor for:

- Compression therapy could potentially restrict the blood flow to the distal portion of the extremity, ultimately causing tissue death, necrosis, and amputation. The skin color should be noted and reported if blue or pale. The patient should be aware of the need to report any numbness, tingling, excess warmth, or coldness in extremities during compression therapy.
- In those with cardiac disease, the fluid shift that occurs with controlling edema may cause cardiac failure and/or pulmonary edema, so patients must note increasing dyspnea, cough, or chest pain.
- Constriction caused by a bandage or compressive garment can restrict movement and cause contractions and skin trauma.
- Displacement of fluid may cause congestion proximal to the compressed legs, so the patient must report any swelling of the knee, thigh, or abdomen.
- Some people may develop sensitivity to materials in the compression material, resulting in itching and rash.

Wound Irrigation at Home

Personal Precautions to Take During Wound Cleansing Irrigations

Wound irrigation should be done in a small room with the doors closed, but not the bathroom. The patient should be seated comfortably or lying down, depending upon the site of the wound. The patient and/or caregiver should wash hands, apply clean gloves, and wear a mask during irrigation. Towels should be placed around the wound area with a basin below the wound to catch the returned solution. The patient should use a squeeze bottle to squirt normal saline on the wound to cleanse drainage and necrotic material, using care to avoid touching the wound with the irrigation tip or disturbing the wound. After irrigation, the hands should be washed and regloved and the wound dressed. The basin should be emptied in the toilet and towels washed. Surfaces in the room should be wiped with a disinfectant. The squeeze bottle and basin should be washed with hot soapy water, rinsed with bleach solution and hot water, then dried and covered with a clean towel until the next use.

Making Saline Irrigating Fluid in the Home Setting

If the patient needs to use a quantity of normal saline to cleanse a wound by irrigation in the home setting, it may be advisable to make normal saline from boiled tap water and salt. A pot and quart glass jar or plastic container and lid should be washed with hot water, rinsed with diluted bleach water and then hot water, and dried (or a jar and lid can be boiled as for canning). Bring a quart of tap water to boil in the pot and keep it boiling for 5 minutes. Add two teaspoons of non-iodized salt and stir until dissolved. The solution should be allowed to cool completely before use. It can be stored in the clean covered glass or plastic container at room temperature and used for up to one week, after which it should be discarded.

Avoiding Wound Infections in the Home

Patients should be aware of the need to avoid illness and infection when they have a healing wound and should take steps to prevent wound infections:

- Visitors should be screened for illness and advised to visit with the patient by phone until well.
- Family members who are ill should not be near the patient or prepare food for them.
- Those with coughs should wear a mask or should cover the mouth with a tissue and remain at least 3 feet from the patient.
- Patient and family should practice good hygiene and good handwashing techniques.
- Wound care procedures should be followed, and contaminated dressing supplies and outdated irrigation solutions discarded.
- Wound care, such as dressing changes, should be done in a clean environment.
- Pets should be groomed regularly and prevented from licking the wound area.

Reinforcing Seating and Turning Schedules

The care provider should reinforce seating and turning schedules when educating the patient:

- Teach methods of turning and positioning the patient every 1-2 hours.
- Draw a clock face to post in the home to remind them to turn the patient, writing the position at the corresponding time on the clock. Time in a chair or in another upright position can be scheduled in the morning for AM care and at mealtimes, with side-lying and supine positioning in between. An alarm clock or timer can also help the patient and caregiver to remember to change position.
- Teach the 8 positions to use: supine with the knees elevated, supine tilted 30 degrees to the right or left, supine with a slight tilt off one sacral side, supine with the head elevated 30 degrees, and prone tilted 30 degrees to either side.
- Stress the prevention of skin breakdown and the fact that positioning is one of the most important components of prevention, along with nutrition, hydration, support surfaces, and cleaning and drying the skin after elimination.

Skin Temperature Monitoring in the Home

Temperature monitoring is a way to make early identification of areas of the foot that are experiencing tissue stress. This method uses special foot thermometers to identify compromised areas before subtle surface signs can be detected by the patient or caregiver. It is invaluable for patients who are at high risk for skin ulceration. The patient and caregiver are given a foot diagram with areas of the foot to be tested, including those that are problematic for this individual. They are instructed to let the bare foot come to room temperature for 5 or 10 minutes before testing. Temperature is then recorded on the diagram for each circled area. The time and date are also recorded. Temperature elevations of 3 degrees over the baseline obtained in the physician's office should be reported. The patient can also be taught measures to take when this occurs to provide immediate relief of pressure to the area. Serial temperature measurements can then be taken to see if these measures are working.

Managing Incontinence to Prevent Skin Breakdown

Prompt cleaning after incontinence removes irritating urea and enzymes from the skin. The skin should be washed with soap and water or pre-moistened wipes. The area must then be dried thoroughly. A lubricating cream, such as zinc oxide, helps to protect the perineal areas. The patient may wear disposable briefs or use bed pads. Disposable adult briefs wick fluid away from the skin, but should be changed when wet. Scheduled toileting every 1 ½ or 2 hours, after meals, and before bedtime can decrease incontinence from occurring. Fluids should not be withheld to decrease incontinence because dehydration further compromises skin. Male external condom catheters may be used with a small leg collection bag. The condom must be removed for hygiene and to inspect skin on a regular basis. Stool softeners or fiber may help to regulate bowel movements.

Types of Moisturizers

Patients should be provided information about the different types of moisturizers in order to make the best for their skin. Moisturizing helps hydrate the skin, prevent dryness and cracking, and skin breakdown. It should be done after bathing and other times during the day. There are primarily 3 types although there are many varieties. Patients should use hypoallergenic moisturizers without added fragrance:

- **Lotions** contain a lot of water and must be applied often during the day.
- **Creams** contain water and oil and need to be rubbed into the skin 4 times daily.
- **Ointments** often consist of a petrolatum or lanolin combined with the least amount of water. They provide a protective layer over the skin that holds in moisture. They have the longest lasting moisturizing action of all three although they may be occlusive.

Encouraging Smoking Cessation

Smoking directly affects vascular functioning, and patients must be encouraged to stop smoking in order to experience proper wound healing.

Methods

Methods to encourage a patient to stop smoking:

- Discuss the social effects of smoking and the patient's feelings about smoking.
- List ways that smoking harms not only the patient but also family members and pets.
- Stress the use of smoking cessation aids and sources of support so that the patient doesn't feel that he or she must quit without help.
- Refer the patient to sources for free nicotine patches and tips on quitting.
- Enlist family members for support and encouragement.
- Teach the patient and family how smoking affects the patient's vascular problems, causing a high risk of wounds, ulcers, and poor healing.
- Help the patient to devise rewards at regular intervals for quitting.
- Enlist the aid of the physician as needed for pulmonary function testing, medications to use for cessation, and added encouragement and support with each clinic visit.

Nicotine Replacement Therapy

Nicotine replacement therapy (NRT) can increase the success of smoking cessation. Nicotine replacement is available in the form of an inhaler or nasal spray by prescription. It is also available over-the-counter in the form of gum, patches, and lozenges. The cost of replacement therapy is about the same as the daily cost of cigarettes, depending on the amount and type of nicotine replacement. Use of NRT will help the patient to avoid nicotine withdrawal symptoms such as tension and irritability, drowsiness, and problems with concentration. However, there can be side effects from NRT, including heartburn, hiccups, skin irritation from the patches, vertigo, tachycardia, sleeplessness, nausea, vomiting, aching muscles, and stiffness. Patients should be advised to consult with the physician before using nicotine replacement products. NRT should not be used when the patient is pregnant. Identify non-nicotine medications that can help the patient quit smoking.

Nicotine Patches

Nicotine patches require three hours for the drug to be absorbed through the skin into the blood stream. Some patches are designed to be worn during waking hours and some for 24 hours. There are different strengths available for light and heavy smokers. Each patch contains an adhesive that causes it to adhere to the skin. The nicotine patch can cause skin irritation and may not adhere in humid weather or when the patient perspires heavily. The patch should be changed at the same time daily to keep the nicotine level in the blood at a constant state. The old patch should be discarded carefully by folding it and placing it in the trash so that children and pets are not able to access it. The patient should not use patches if they continue to smoke as this increases blood levels of nicotine.

Nicotine Spray or Inhaler

The use of a nicotine spray or an inhaler as aids for smoking cessation:

- **Nicotine nasal spray** is absorbed rapidly through the nasal mucosa. The patient should deliver 2 sprays into each nostril up to 5 times per hour. Side effects include nose and throat irritation. Heavy smokers may succeed with this form of NRT since it reaches the bloodstream more quickly than other NRT.
- **The nicotine inhaler** uses cartridges of nicotine vapor that the patient puffs on for 20 minutes up to 16 times a day. Side effects are mouth and throat irritation and a cough, which decreases over time.

Both methods should be used consistently for effectiveness; however, they are more expensive to use than nicotine gum, patches, or lozenges.

Nicotine Gum and Lozenges

Patients should stop smoking when gum or lozenge therapy begins. Enough should be used to reduce craving and withdrawal symptoms, especially in the beginning. Patients should not eat or drink for 15 minutes prior to or while chewing the gum or using lozenges. Side effects are irritation of the mouth, throat, and gums. The gum is dense and may damage dental work. Both gum and lozenges should be disposed of safely out of the reach of children and pets. Both come in 2 mg and 4 mg strengths:

- **Nicotine gum** is chewed until tingling is felt, and then the gum should be parked between the gum and cheek. When the tingling sensation decreases, the gum is chewed a few times and parked again. This continues until the gum no longer produces the tingling sensation, and then it is discarded.
- **Nicotine lozenges** should dissolve slowly and must not be chewed or swallowed or heartburn and nausea may occur.

Non-Nicotine Medications That Help Patients Quit Smoking

Non-nicotine medications that help the patient quit smoking:

- **Zyban** (bupropion hydrochloride) has been used since 1977. It is also an antidepressant. The patient begins taking Zyban a week prior to quitting. During this time the drug begins to reach a stable level in the blood and the smoker will notice that cigarettes do not taste as good and are not as satisfying. Zyban helps to remove the urge to smoke but its exact action is unknown. Side effects include dry mouth, dizziness, and insomnia. It should be taken for 12 weeks to help the patient establish smoke-free behavior before stopping the drug.
- **Chantix** (varenicline) is a new drug that partially blocks nicotine receptors. It also reduces the pleasure of smoking while reducing side effects of nicotine withdrawal. It can be taken for 12 to 24 weeks. Side effects include nausea, vomiting, headache, flatus, insomnia, abnormal dreaming, and altered taste.

Self-Care for Venous Insufficiency

Venous insufficiency is a condition that occurs when the venous wall or valves in the leg veins are not working effectively, making it difficult for blood to return to the heart from the legs.

Points to teach the patient about self-care for venous insufficiency:

- Teach the patient about the disease, symptoms, and personal risk factors to modify, including smoking.
- Explain the reason for compression therapy and how to apply stockings properly.
- Teach skin assessment and care for the legs and feet. The patient should inspect the skin daily for any signs of trauma, redness, pain, or skin ulcer formation. Lubricants or emollients should be applied to the legs and feet at night to counteract the drying effect of compression stockings. The patient should learn to avoid crossing the legs and to elevate the legs when sitting several times a day.
- Stress the need to avoid injury to the skin of the legs and feet.
- Counsel the patient on improving nutritional intake.

Self-Care for Arterial Insufficiency

Arterial insufficiency is any condition that slows or stops the flow of blood through the arteries, such as atherosclerosis.

Points to remember when teaching the patient about self-care for arterial insufficiency:

- Teach the patient the pathophysiology behind arterial insufficiency: hypertension, diabetes, and high cholesterol, signs and symptoms of these diseases, and personal risk factors that can be modified, including smoking and diet.
- Be sure the patient understands doctor's orders, including activity limitations and medications.
- Teach the daily inspection of the legs and feet to check for symptoms to report, such as redness, skin breakdown, and pain.
- Teach skin and toenail care, including washing and drying of the legs and feet, application of emollients, and filing of the nails straight across.
- Warn against going barefooted and review the proper fit for shoes and socks.
- Caution the patient to check bath temperature to avoid burning by bath water that is too hot.

Management of Immunosuppression

Immunosuppression may be the result of co-morbid conditions, such as AIDS, or medications, such as chemotherapy or steroids. Immunosuppression can decrease wound healing and increase the incidence of infection because the body can't destroy pathogenic agents through normal defense mechanisms. Careful management of immunosuppression is critical to healing:

- **Adjust dosages** or discontinue medications contributing to immunosuppression if possible, including steroid avoidance or steroid withdrawal regimens.
- **Monitor wound condition** carefully for changes or lack of healing response that may indicate infection because infection is the most common result of immunosuppression and may not be accompanied by increase of temperature or other usual indications.
- **Monitor immune status** with regular blood tests to determine changes.
- **Provide antimicrobials** as indicated prophylactically to prevent wound infections.
- **Maintain clean environment** and ensure staff use standard precautions.
- Observe for opportunistic infections, such as candidiasis.

EDUCATION FOR DIABETICS

GENERAL MANAGEMENT

Management of diabetes and maintaining glucose control for both Type I (insulin-dependent) and Type II diabetes may be the important determinant of the ability of the wound to heal. Plans should be individualized but usually include the following:

- **Establish goals**: HbA1c level of 6.5% or lower.
- **Maintain normal glycemic levels** during healing:
  - Monitor glucose 4 times daily up to every 4 hours.
  - Type I: Monitor food and insulin intake, adjusting as needed.
  - Type II: Focus on diet, medical control, weight loss, and maintenance of weight loss.
  - Avoid or limit use of alcohol because of unpredictable effects on glucose.
- **Institute exercise program**:
  - Type I: Increases general health and well-being.
  - Type II: Decreases insulin resistance.
- **Treat co-morbid conditions**, such as atherosclerosis, hypertension, and early renal disease.
- **Cease smoking**, which interferes with circulation and damages vasculature.
- **Make lifestyle changes** that will promote long-term glucose control.

INFORMATION CONCERNING DIABETIC NEUROPATHY

The patient should be urged to contact the physician if signs of diabetic neuropathy, such as altered sensation, is detected in the lower extremities, including sensations of tingling, bugs crawling on the skin, burning, or numbness. The neuropathic foot can't adjust to painful areas with each step. The loss of sensation and pain makes injuries harder to detect, so the importance of daily checking the feet must be stressed. Motor neuropathy results in muscular, bone, and joint deformities. The loss of autonomic control causes the skin to become dry, scaly, and to crack from lack of nutrients and hydration. The presence of neuropathy greatly increases the risk of foot trauma so this patient must be extra vigilant. Neuropathy often leads to ulcerations that are deep and hard to heal. Rubbing from improperly fitted footwear, pressure on the bottom of the foot that isn't relieved, and injury from trauma are the main causes of foot ulcers and problems in this population.

PROPER SKIN-CARE TIPS

The diabetic should be taught to report skin problems as soon as possible, since there is a decreased ability to fight infections. Blood glucose should be regulated to help prevent dryness. The skin, especially skin folds and the feet, should be checked daily when bathing or undressing, and baths and showers should be less frequent, especially in the winter months. Baths should be warm, but not hot enough to burn skin. Only fragrance-free moisturizing soaps and mild shampoos should be used. Moisturizers that consist of a mixture of oil and water (such as Lubriderm or Alpha-Keri) should be used frequently to prevent dry, itchy skin, but not between toes to avoid fungal growth. Scratching damages skin and must be avoided. Powders may be helpful in areas where skin rubs together. Women should not use deodorant sprays in the vaginal area. Humidity in the home should be increased, especially in the winter months. Patients should not be hesitant to contact their physician, podiatrist, or dermatologist about any problem areas on the skin.

Risk of Foot Ulcers for Patients with Diabetes

One should motivate diabetic patients to learn foot care by explaining their risks for foot problems. Patients should be taught that diabetes commonly causes foot and leg amputation in the diabetic patient but may be avoided with proper care. Foot ulcers and trauma are the cause for hospitalization in up to 25% of all diabetic admissions. Diabetics are up to 46% more likely to need an amputation, and if one is needed, another amputation on the same or opposite extremity is more likely. Survival up to five years after an amputation is 70% or below. Hispanics, African-Americans, and Native Americans have the highest amputation rates. The patient should be advised to see a podiatrist as needed. The importance of maintaining blood glucose control through diet, medication, and exercise to reduce risk factors for foot ulcers should be stressed.

Frequency of Podiatry Visits

Podiatrists inspect the feet and identify areas that need treatment or offloading to prevent ulcer formation. They treat calluses and trim thick or problem nails:

- The patient without altered sensation should be seen by a podiatrist yearly to ensure continued foot health.
- When nails are not ingrown, tented, or thick, the patient can use an emery board to keep them trim.
- The patient who has impaired sensation needs to have podiatry care at least twice a year. During this visit the patient can be advised on the type of shoes needed to ensure proper fitting and pressure relief as needed.
- A patient with neuropathy who also has another problem, such as decreased circulation or bony deformity, should be seen every 2 or 3 months and fitted with therapeutic shoes.
- A high-risk patient who has healed ulcers, a previous amputation, or nail problems needs to be seen by a podiatrist every 1 to 2 months to monitor conditions and for nail care.

Shoes for Patients with Diabetes or Foot Problems

Any patient with diabetes or foot problems should be counseled to always wear shoes and not go barefoot to prevent trauma:

- Off the shelf shoes must be deep enough to accommodate deformed toes or other areas. They should be made of soft leather without stitching that will conform to foot shape and retain that shape. Shoes should allow space for an insole that can be modified to relieve pressure in troublesome areas on the bottom of the foot without redistributing pressure to the top of the foot.
- Patients should be taught how to trim insoles to provide off-loading to problem areas. If shoes or insoles are modified, the patient must monitor other areas for problems that can occur when windows are cut into shoes or insoles.
- Patients that must have custom-made shoes or orthotics should wear them at all times for walking. Patients should maintain shoes and insoles and replace them when worn.
- Patients who have Medicare Part B should be evaluated to determine eligibility for Medicare payment for shoes and inserts.

Socks for Patients with Diabetes or Foot Problems

Patients with foot problems should be taught to buy socks without seams over the toes that can cause friction. Tube socks do not work because there are always folds formed that cause pressure and restriction. Socks should be replaced if they are worn out, not mended. They should be made of as much cotton as possible to absorb perspiration. They should fit well without extra material at the toes or heels and should fit smoothly across the top of the foot. Cushioned socks are best. Socks should not have a tight top that restricts circulation. Specialty socks with silicone padding or custom-made socks that fit a partial foot may be required. These socks may enclose each toe to decrease moisture. Two thin socks should be worn to break in new shoes to allow movement between the socks to avoid shearing pressure and blistering.

Teaching Diabetic Foot Care to Caregivers

Patients who are unable to inspect and care for their feet should have caregivers who can be taught to assume this duty:

- Patients who are obese or have mobility problems may not be able to get the feet into a position in which all areas can be inspected.
- Patients with visual problems need to have their feet inspected by others.
- Patients with cognitive problems, such as Alzheimer's disease, may lack adequate comprehension to manage skin care and need to have their skin care needs met by others as well.

Caregivers should be taught all aspects of foot and skin care and be willing to assume this responsibility. They should be encouraged to accompany the patients to physician and podiatrist visits so that ongoing education can be provided.

Exercise Practices

The patient with neuropathy or other foot problems should be taught that walking causes 150% of the person's weight to rest on the foot with each step and jogging increases this to 300%. Therefore, the patient should not jog but should walk with slow, short steps only as needed and not for exercise. Appropriate exercise for these patients can include specialized low-impact aerobics and dance if appropriate. **Exercise** that is less stressful to the feet includes chair and mat exercises, swimming, or cycling. Isometric exercises can help to maintain muscle strength and can be done without weight bearing. The patient must be instructed to wear shoes while exercising and soft pool shoes when swimming to avoid injuries. The feet should be dried well after swimming.

Barriers to Caring for Wounds

Financial and psychosocial barriers to preventing and caring for wounds include:

- Low income, lack of insurance and resources, fear of being unable to provide for the self and/or family
- Inadequate diet and nutrition
- Lack of health literacy, illiteracy
- Lack of transportation options to healthcare providers (no auto, no public transportation, inability to afford options), distance from healthcare providers (such as in rural areas).
- Fear of doctors, phobias (needles, hospitals)
- Mental illness (bipolar, schizophrenia, depression), stress
- Religious beliefs (Christian Scientist, Jehovah Witness), cultural differences (including language)
- Lack of adequate housing, homelessness, unsanitary conditions
- Lack of family/friend emotional support
- Inadequate communication/coordination among healthcare providers
- Substance abuse, drug and/or alcohol use
- Threat to job security if absent from work
- Low expectation of recovery, perception of unfair treatment, uncaring healthcare provider
- Dysfunctional interpersonal relationships (friends, family, caregivers)
- Inadequate instructions for follow-up

Patient Adherence

Patient Adherence to Wound Care and Wound Prevention

If a wound is to heal and close, then patient adherence to wound care and preventive measures is a critical element. Patients who have had previous negative experiences, who lack support systems, who don't understand what they need to do, and who have lifestyle risks (homelessness, substance abuse, smoking) are especially at risk for nonadherence. Elements of the task may also affect adherence: complex tasks, inability to carry out the tasks, and aversion to the task because of pain or discomfort.

Methods to ensure adherence include:

- Provide step by step instructions and allow ample practice time.
- Provide emotional support and positive feedback when appropriate.
- Apprise the patient of progress, using pictures and/or diagrams.
- Encourage the patient to express feelings.
- Note early signs of nonadherence but avoid being judgmental: "I see that you weren't able to change the dressings every day."
- Provide continuity of care to allow the patient to establish a relationship with caregiver.

Encouraging Patient Compliance with Wound Care Regimen

Methods to encourage patient compliance with wound care regimen:

- Take care to assess how the wound care regimen affects the patient.
- Refer to a social worker to help find resources to meet financial obligations and pay for medications, dressings, food, and bills.
- Assist to get help with ADLs, housekeeping, and other needs. This will help the patient feel that he or she can take the time from other obligations to heal.
- Teach about the healing process and how the wound care regimen encourages healing in the shortest time possible.
- Point out even minor improvements in the wound or ulcer to give them hope and encouragement to continue the regime. Keeping a wound progress chart can show tangible evidence of progress.
- Help establish realistic goals and enlist family members to help remind the patient of the goals and the ways to obtain them.
- Assess patient and family coping with each visit and teach as needed to help encourage compliance.

Common Behaviors in Patients with Wounds

There is a wide range of behavior in patients with wounds:

- Some become deeply concerned about the wound and are motivated to learn about its cause, healing processes, and treatment. They maintain control by taking an active role in caring for the wound.
- Some react with denial and refuse to cooperate, sometimes worsening their condition by continuing, for example, to walk on an ulcerated foot.
- Some become belligerent and angry and lash out at family and caregivers.
- Some become depressed and withdrawn and may do nothing or react passively.
- Some say one thing and do another; for example, patients may state they have quit smoking while continuing to do so.
- Some set a goal for the healing to be completed, such as a social event that encourages them to learn and be compliant with treatment.
- Some patients may enjoy the attention and seek to continue getting this attention when the wound is healed.

Psychosocial Factors Affecting Care

Psychosocial factors affecting care include:

- **Ability to learn/perform care**: Cognitive impairment and hearing or vision deficits may interfere with the ability to learn, especially if appropriate educational materials are not available. Physical disabilities may make it difficult for patients to learn or perform some aspects of care. Language differences may result in impaired comprehension.
- **Economic implications**: Patients and families may be severely impacted if the wage earner is unable to continue to work or if they lack the resources (insurance, financial) to pay for needed care.
- **Education**: Patients may lack an adequate educational background to understand the implications of disease, to read materials, and to follow directions. Health literacy may be very low, so patients may have misconceptions about disease.
- **Mental status**: Patients often experience increased stress associated with illness, and this may interfere with functioning. Mental impairment may impact a patient's ability to participate in care. Additionally, depression is common, especially with chronic illness, and may cause patients to withdraw or fail to comply with treatment.

Patient Safety

Performing Patient Transfer From Chair to Bed

Transferring a patient from chair to bed consists of the following steps:

1. Apply bed brakes and place the bed in the lowest position. A lift sheet should be on the bed.
2. Place the wheelchair next to the bed so the patient moves toward the stronger side if one side of the body is weak.
3. Lock brakes and remove the footrests.
4. Place a gait belt around the patient's waist.
5. Be sure the belt is not placed over a female patient's breasts.
6. Instruct the patient to push down on the arms of the chair if able to while standing up.
7. Perform a stand-pivot-transfer.
8. Seat the patient on the bed as far back as possible.
9. Help the patient turn onto the bed by lifting the legs as the patient turns.
10. Instruct the patient to press down on the bed during the turn to help prevent friction on the buttocks.
11. Two people should use the lift sheet to hoist the patient to the proper position in the middle of the bed.

Performing Patient Transfer From Chair to Chair

When transferring a patient from chair to chair, first instruct the patient in the transfer procedure. Position the chair that the patient is to be transferred to in a position that is slightly oblique to the first chair and lock the brakes if either chair is a wheelchair. The patient should be moving toward the strong side if one side of the body is weak:

1. Remove the footrests from the wheelchair.
2. Place a gait belt around the patient's waist.
3. Be sure that the belt is not placed over a female patient's breasts.
4. Instruct the patient to push down on the arms of the chair if able to while standing up.
5. Perform a stand-pivot-transfer.
6. Instruct the patient to reach down to grasp the arms of the chair as you help him or her sit.
7. Help the patient to readjust position until seated properly in the chair.
8. Reapply footrests to the wheelchair and position them so that the thighs are in a 90° angle to the body.
9. If the patient is paraplegic, use two people to accomplish the transfer.

Performing Patient Transfer From Bed to Stretcher

The following are steps for patient transfer from bed to stretcher:

1. Lower the side rails of the bed and lock the brakes.
2. Place the stretcher next to the bed and lock its brakes as well.
3. Raise the bed to the level of the stretcher.
4. While the patient is lying supine, instruct him/her to place the arms across the body.
5. One person should be next to the bed and two people should be on the outside of the stretcher.
6. On the count of three, all three people should lift the sheet slightly as the two next to the stretcher pull the patient across the gap and onto the middle of the stretcher.
7. Place a pillow under the patient's head and cover with a blanket.
8. Raise the head of the stretcher to a comfortable level.
9. Raise the side rails of the stretcher, unlock the wheels, and transport the patient.

Evidence Based Practice

Evidence-Based Research and Wound Care

For many years, common practice was accepted as evidence of effectiveness with little or no research to support or refute the perception; however, since the 1970s, when Archie Cochrane first advocated the need for research to support practice, evidence-based research has become one of the primary change agents in the practice of medicine. Evidence-based research provides information about the most successful approaches to wound care and also provides information about the areas of wound care that need further research. As part of evidence-based research, the researcher should review the current literature that is reliable and relevant, such as juried journals and collections, such as the Cochrane Collaboration, which provides metanalysis of similar studies to determine the most reliable information regarding outcomes. Relevant journals include *Advances in Wound Care; Journal of Wound Care; Advances in Skin & Wound Care; International Wound Journal; Journal of Wound, Ostomy, and Continence Nursing; Ostomy Wound Management;* and *The International Journal of Lower Extremity Wounds.* An online resource for peer-reviewed information is *World Wide Wounds.*

Levels of Evidence

Levels of evidence are categorized according to the scientific evidence available to support the recommendations, as well as existing state and federal laws. While recommendations are voluntary, they are often used as a basis for state and federal regulations:

- **Category IA** is well supported by evidence from experimental, clinical, or epidemiologic studies and is strongly recommended for implementation.
- **Category IB** has supporting evidence from some studies, has a good theoretical basis, and is strongly recommended for implementation.
- **Category IC** is required by state or federal regulations or is an industry standard.
- **Category II** is supported by suggestive clinical or epidemiologic studies, has a theoretical basis, and is suggested for implementation.
- **Category III** is supported by descriptive studies (such as comparisons, correlations, and case studies) and may be useful.
- **Category IV** is obtained from expert opinion or authorities only.
- **Unresolved** means there is no recommendation because of a lack of consensus or evidence.

Research Methods for Wound Care Practice

Various research methods can be applied to wound care practice. However, wound care practices should be based on evidence-based research already conducted as there must be justification for the interventions chosen. Clear definitions should be developed for inclusion, exclusion, and eligibility criteria, and guidelines for care should be outlined. **Methodologies**:

- Randomized controlled trial comparing different approaches to wound care.
- Blind randomized assessment of initial and final wound photographs: This type of research is done after-the-fact but assessment must have clear criteria because subjective evaluations may vary.
- Standardization of treatment so that all healthcare providers utilize the same steps and criteria for assessment, such as assessment by digital measurement, to determine if this makes a difference in outcomes.
- Comparing digital measurements with standard measurements to determine accuracy.
- Molecular level research utilizing tissue samples.
- Observational studies may include cohort studies, case-control studies, matched studies, and cross-sectional studies.

Multidisciplinary Teams

Multidisciplinary Teams

A multidisciplinary team is comprised of experts in a number of different fields, collaborating to address the complex problems associated with wound care and underlying pathology. Instead of the serial approach to problem-solving involved in the traditional model of care, where referrals are made in response to problems that arise with little communication among specialists, the multidisciplinary approach is to identify potential problems and institute preventive measures at their onset, with all members communicating and sharing information. Responsibilities of the wound care team include:

- **Prevention**: Establish standard risk assessment protocols and formulary. Incorporate national prevention guidelines.
- **Treatment**: Establish clinical protocols and product formularies in relation to national treatment practice guidelines.
- **Documentation**: Provide standardized methods.
- **Education**: Provide literature/training for patients and staff.
- **Quality Management**: Evaluate outcomes and disseminate findings.
- **Research**: Conduct clinical trials.
- **Care conferences**: Create individualized care plans.

Advantages

A team of individuals with expertise in wound care brings a combination of years of experience and skill to the patient's bedside. They use this skill to assess the wound and determine the range of treatments and dressings that would be effective. They consider the cost of the supplies and the patient's individual health, emotional status, and financial status when choosing treatments that will accomplish the goal of healing. The team may designate staff nurses to carry out treatments and assess the wound on a weekly and PRN (as needed) basis to evaluate the efficacy of treatment and to document wound progress. The team is able to evaluate progress consistently using the same people to assess wounds week after week. The team can also spot facility-wide needs in terms of skin trauma prevention, propose changes in techniques, procedures, and equipment, and evaluate the improvements. They can do research to determine new treatments available and do trials on wound care methods in the facility, contributing to evidence-based care.

Indications for Referrals to Specialists

Various specialists may be indicated for referral in the care of specific patients:

- **Occupational therapist**: Patients with weakness, disability, or impairments may need OT to assist them in carrying out ADLs and IADLs and finding and using appropriate assistive devices.
- **Physical therapist**: Patients with physical weakness or disability may need PT to maintain or improve strength and mobility and to prevent further deterioration.
- **Nutritionist**: Patients may need nutritional guidance to ensure an adequate diet to meet specific needs, such as high protein diets for wound healing and low-calorie diets for obesity.
- **Diabetes educator**: Diabetic patients are at risk of multiple complications, so information about disease, diet, medications, lifestyle choices, foot/skin care, and preventive measures is critical.
- **Podiatrist**: Patients with poor mobility or vision, especially diabetics, should see podiatrists for routine nail trimming and foot care to prevent problems.
- **Dermatologist**: Patients with rashes or skin lesions need to be examined and treated and may need periodic skin checks.
- **Case manager**: The case manager serves as a resource for clients with multiple or chronic health problems and provides information to help them to make care decisions, to obtain healthcare services, and to achieve quality outcomes.

Referrals for Medical/Surgical Interventions

Referrals for medical surgical interventions are an important part of wound care as healing requires that medical conditions be monitored carefully and treated, especially such disorders as diabetes and peripheral vascular disease, but this is also true of almost all acute or chronic disorders. Conditions that were stable prior to wound development may deteriorate or change in character in response to the body's needs during healing or infections that may occur. Patients may require referrals, such as to endocrinologists or infectious disease specialists. Wounds with extensive eschar may require surgical debridement in order to promote healing. It is important that the patient be an integral member of any planning and discussion. The patient must be apprised of the reasons for referrals and the types of testing, care, and procedures that will be done to ensure cooperation and to alleviate the patient's fears and anxiety.

Handoff/Transition of Patients with Wounds

When a patient with a wound is to be transferred, such as to a different department, a different level of care, a different facility, or to the patient's home, **handoff/transition** should include complete documentation and verbal communication regarding:

- Demographic information, such as name, diagnoses, address, and telephone number
- List of medications and treatments
- Equipment/supplies needed for care
- Teaching strategies utilized with patient/caregiver and response
- Consultations/referrals, such as to social workers of specialists
- Follow-up needed, such as appointments and rehabilitation
- Documentation of all wounds, including discussion of location, size, depth, induration, drainage, granulation, infection, eschar, tunneling, and abscesses
- Notation of any high-risk pressure areas
- Explanation of all past and current approaches to wound therapies and patient/caregiver response
- Explanation of all past and current approaches to wound prevention (positioning, seat cushions, air mattresses and response)
- Psychosocial barriers to care or compliance, such as cognitive impairment, physical disabilities, poverty, and lack of support system
- Nutritional guidelines (high protein) to promote healing

Legal Concepts

Protecting Patient's Privacy During Wound Care

Wound care should be done in a private area so others cannot observe the treatment. The room should have a door and a curtain around the bed area. One should always knock and wait for permission prior to entering the room or going behind a drawn curtain. When providing wound care, one should uncover only the part of body being treated, keeping the rest of the body covered and warm. Other people should not be in the room unless assistance is needed for the wound care, and the wound should not be discussed with others in the room without including the patient in the discussion. Schedules for turning or other wound care should not be posted in public areas. If the patient has visitors, one must not detail wound care or discuss other private healthcare matters with the patient in front of them.

Standard of Care Requirements for Discovery of a Pressure Injury

Upon discovery of a pressure injury, the actions of the facility and its providers are judged against a standard of care to determine liability. Swift action according to policy is the best defense:

- Measure and document the injury, including staging if possible.
- Conduct a pain assessment.
- Take action to dress the wound and take pressure off the area.
- Document physician notification, the response, and orders given.
- Clarify that the physician will notify the family.
- Implement treatment measures promptly and document them.
- Make referrals if needed to evaluate nutrition and hydration status or to do vascular studies.
- Add the new problems and interventions to the patient care plan.
- Consistently document the treatments, dressing changes, and wound status on a form and in narrative notes in one place on the chart.

Legal Requirements for Pressure Injury Prevention

A facility can be held liable for failure to prevent pressure injuries. There must be an effort to assess the patient for risk factors for skin breakdown at admission. When risk is found, the physician must be notified and treatment or preventive measures must be taken. Those measures must be evaluated for efficacy in prevention of breakdown and changed as needed. All interventions for risk factors must be incorporated in the patient's care plan and documentation must show that all interventions were employed as written. Pressure injuries can still develop on patients who are critically ill in spite of these measures, but when the facility can prove that preventive measures were routinely taken, they are not held liable. Medicare does not assign a higher-paying DRG for pressure injuries unless they were already evident on admission. Any organization that deviates from state or federal regulations related to prevention of pressure injuries may be legally liable.

Time Out Procedure

A time out must occur just prior to a procedure, such as an incision or puncture of the skin of a patient or an insertion of a foreign body into the patient's body. During the time out, the participants in the procedure verify that it is the right patient and right procedure on the right portion of the body. Patient position is checked and the proper equipment and implants are verified for the procedure. Time out takes place in the room where the procedure is to be performed. This time out must be documented in the patient's record, including the names of the entire team who participate in the time out. The Joint Commission mandates the time out as part of the process developed to prevent medical errors. The other two steps in this process are pre-operative verification and marking of the correct portion of the body prior to the procedure. Time outs are NOT required before a venipuncture, urinary catheter insertion, or NG tube insertion.

Certification and Government Regulations

Wound Care Certification

Wound Care Certification is available to licensed healthcare professionals, including those with an RN, LVN/LPN, PA, PT, PTA, OT, OTA, MD, DO, or DPM license, who meet both an education requirement and an experience requirement:

- **Education**: Either graduations from a skin/wound management educational program that meets certification criteria OR current active CWCN, CWON, CWOCN or CWS certification.
- **Experience**: Either 120 hours of hands-on clinical training with an approved preceptor (NAWCO) OR 2 years fulltime/4 years part-time experience in wound care, management, education, or research.

Applicants must pay a fee and pass the WCC certification exam. To renew the certification, the person must have a license in good standing, a current unexpired certification, and have completed 60 contact hours of approved continuing education in wound care in the previous 5 years. As with other licensed personnel, the scope of practice is determined by the state practice act appropriate to the discipline and duties may be further determined by the employing agency and job description.

Certified Wound Specialist

A Certified Wound Specialist is a licensed medical professional (OD, DPM, MD, NP, PA, PT, OT, PharmD, RD, or RN) with three or more years clinical experience working in wound care or one year of a fellowship in wound care. Candidates should have master level training in the management of wounds. While no specific wound care program is outlined, the candidate must submit documents detailing clinical experience as well as letters of recommendation. The candidate must also pass the certification examination if the clinical experience is accepted and the candidate is deemed eligible for certification. The CWS must renew certification annually by paying a fee and submitting proof of six hours of continuing education in wound care. The scope of practice may vary from state to state because it is determined by the state(s) in which the person is licensed to practice and the type of licensure. The CWS must retake the qualifying exam every 10 years.

Government Regulations Pertaining to Wound Care

Various government regulations pertaining to wound care management relate to licensure, who is allowed to provide wound care, price-setting (which may be based on outcomes), and quality measures. Regulatory bodies include OSHA (safety issues, infection control), the FDA (drugs and medical devices), and CMS (standards and reimbursement) as well as state boards of nursing, physical therapy, medicine, and osteopathy (scope of practice), but other organizations, such as the Joint Commission, WOCN society, and AAWC, provide rules and guidelines. CMS (Medicare, Medicaid) has a primary role in setting regulations that effect the entire medical and insurance industries. Reimbursement in most cases is now directly tied to the quality of care and to progress in wound healing. This has resulted in increased focus on accurate documentation and better methods of assessing and treating wounds in order to improve outcomes. Medicare regulations are consistent, although different types of facilities have different methods of reimbursement. Medicaid programs vary from one state to another, so the way in which wound care is reimbursed may also vary.

Medicare's Therapeutic Shoe Bill

Ill-fitting or stylish shoes may cause too much pressure on bony prominences or cause pressure that results in foot ulcers. Diabetic patients with Medicare Part B may be eligible for benefits under Medicare's Therapeutic Shoe Bill, passed by Congress in 1996. It is designed for diabetic patients who have inadequate circulation, foot deformities, calluses, peripheral neuropathy, a previous pre-ulcerative callus or foot ulcer, or an amputation of a portion of the foot or of the entire foot. Once a year, the patient is eligible for a combination of shoe inserts, custom made orthotics, modified depth shoes, or custom-made shoes to meet the individual's need to prevent foot ulceration. A physician, such as a podiatrist, must prescribe the shoes and specific insoles. Patients who are eligible should be informed of what is available to them under this bill to help them preserve their feet.

Wound Care Practice Test

Want to take this practice test in an online interactive format?
Check out the online resources page, which includes interactive practice questions and much more: **mometrix.com/resources719/cwcn**

1. Which of the following extends from a wound under normal tissue and connects two structures, such as the wound and an organ?

a. undermining
b. fistula
c. tunneling
d. abscess

2. A patient has a wound on the right hip with tunneling and fistulae. Which of the following is *MOST* indicative of an abscess formation?

a. increased purulent discharge
b. increased wound pain
c. increased erythema and swelling at wound perimeter
d. erythematous, painful, swollen area 3 cm from wound perimeter

3. Which of the following laboratory tests is the most effective to monitor acute changes in nutritional status?

a. total protein
b. albumin
c. prealbumin
d. transferrin

4. On the eighth day of wound care, granulation tissue is evident about the wound perimeter, and the wound is beginning to contract. The wound is in which of the following phases of healing?

a. proliferation
b. inflammation
c. hemostasis
d. maturation

5. Which of the following is the correct procedure for applying Eutectic Mixture of Local Anesthetics (EMLA Cream) to a wound prior to debridement?

a. apply a thin layer (1/8 inch thick) to the wound for 15 minutes, leaving the wound open
b. apply a thick layer (1/4 inch thick) to the wound, extending 1/2 inch past the wound onto surrounding tissue, and cover with plastic wrap for 20-60 minutes
c. apply a thick layer (1/4 inch thick) to the wound surface only and cover with plastic wrap for 15 minutes
d. apply a thin layer (1/8 inch thick) to the wound surface only and cover with a loose dry dressing for 20-60 minutes

6. When doing a routine dressing change for a healing pressure injury on the right hip, which is the most appropriate cleaning solution?

a. povidone-iodine solution
b. hydrogen peroxide
c. alcohol
d. normal saline

7. Which of the following wound irrigation devices will provide approximately 8 psi in irrigant pressure to the wound surface?

a. 35-mL syringe with 19-gauge Angiocath
b. 250-mL squeeze bottle
c. bulb syringe
d. 6-mL syringe with 19-gauge Angiocath

8. Which of the following is the most important criterion when assessing a patient's level of wound pain?

a. patient's behavior
b. type of wound
c. patient's report of pain
d. patient's facial expression

9. Which of the following is likely to have the *MOST* negative effect on wound healing for a 65-year-old woman?

a. hypoalbuminemia
b. BMI of 20.2
c. BMI of 28
d. vegan diet

10. Which of the following is the most definitive method for obtaining a wound specimen for culture and sensitivities?

a. tissue biopsy
b. sterile swab of wound
c. needle biopsy
d. sterile swab of discharge

11. A patient with an infected abdominal wound is taking a number of drugs. Which of the following is most likely to impair healing?

a. phenytoin
b. corticosteroid
c. prostaglandin
d. estrogen

12. A burn extending into the dermis with obvious blistering would be classified as

a. first degree.
b. second degree.
c. third degree.
d. full thickness.

13. Which of the following results from smoking cigarettes?

a. vasodilation
b. vasoconstriction
c. increased oxygen transport
d. increased oxygen tension

14. When calculating the ankle-brachial index (ABI), if the ankle systolic pressure is 90 mmHg and the brachial systolic pressure is 120 mmHg, what is the ABI?

a. 1.33
b. 13.3
c. 7.5
d. 0.75

15. Using transcutaneous oxygen pressure measurement ($TCPO_2$), which of the following values indicates that oxygenation is adequate for healing?

a. 18 mmHg
b. 20 mmHg
c. 30 mmHg
d. 42 mmHg

16. The method of closure that involves leaving the wound open and allowing it to close naturally through granulation and epithelialization is healing by

a. primary or first intention.
b. secondary or second intention.
c. tertiary or third intention.
d. quaternary prevention.

17. A patient's laboratory results show a serum sodium of 155 mEq/L and a serum osmolality of 300 mOsm/kg. The most likely cause is

a. infection.
b. overhydration.
c. dehydration.
d. malnutrition.

18. Autolytic debridement is most effective for

a. chronic wounds.
b. large burns.
c. small wounds without infection.
d. necrotic wounds.

19. Enzymatic debridement requires application of enzymes

a. 1-2 times daily.
b. 3-4 times daily.
c. 1-2 times weekly.
d. 3-4 times weekly.

20. Which of the following indicates that sharp instrument debridement must be discontinued?

a. purulent discharge occurs
b. black eschar is removed
c. pain and bleeding occur
d. patient complains of fatigue

21. A patient has second and third degree burns on 30% of the body and is in severe pain. Which method of debridement is most indicated?

a. autolytic debridement
b. enzymatic debridement
c. sharp instrument debridement
d. surgical debridement

22. Which method of mechanical debridement may cause damage to granulation tissue and is generally contraindicated?

a. wet-to-dry dressings
b. whirlpool bath
c. irrigation under pressure
d. ultrasound treatment

23. Which of the following topical antimicrobials is most appropriate to treat nasal colonization of *Staphylococcus aureus* in a patient with an open wound?

a. cadexomer iodine
b. metronidazole
c. mupirocin (Bactroban®)
d. silver sulfadiazine

24. Which of the following is a contraindication to negative pressure wound therapy?

a. chronic Stage IV pressure injury
b. wound malignancy
c. unresponsive arterial ulcer
d. dehiscent surgical wound

25. Which of the following is the primary goal in referring a patient for multidisciplinary consultation?

a. prevention of complications
b. treatment of complications
c. education
d. identification of outcomes

26. Becaplermin (Regranex®) gel is indicated for which type of wound?

a. venous stasis ulcer
b. pressure injury
c. sutured/stapled wound
d. diabetic ulcer

27. Which of the following types of dressing is indicated for treatment of a full-thickness infected wound with large amount of exudate?

a. alginate
b. hydrocolloid
c. hydrogel
d. semipermeable film

28. What hyperbaric oxygen therapy (HBOT) treatment regimen is usually recommended for chronic wounds and lower extremity diabetic ulcers?

a. compression at 2 ATA 3 times 60 minutes daily for 48 hours
b. compression at 2.0-2.4 ATA for 90 minutes daily for at least 30 treatments
c. compression at 3 ATA for 2-4 hour periods 3-4 times daily
d. compression at 3.0-3.5 ATA for 60-90 minutes 2 times daily for 2-3 days and then decreasing frequency over 4-6 days

29. Which NPIAP stage is a pressure injury characterized by deep full-thickness ulceration that exposes subcutaneous tissue with possible presence of slough, tunneling, and undermining but without visibility of underlying muscle, tendon, or bone?

a. stage I
b. stage II
c. stage III
d. stage IV

30. What is the most common cause of shear?

a. "sheet burn"
b. elevating the head of the bed >30°
c. lifting the patient with a pull sheet
d. turning the patient side to side

31. What is the minimal thickness of a support surface for a chair?

a. one inch
b. two inches
c. three inches
d. four inches

32. When turning and repositioning patients, what is the preferred position for the patient to reduce pressure?

a. prone
b. supine
c. 30° lateral
d. 90° side-lying

33. On the Braden scale for predicting risk of developing pressure injuries, a patient scores 2 (1 to 4 or 1 to 3 scale) on each of 6 parameters (total score 12). What is the patient's risk of developing a pressure injury?

a. very minimal risk
b. breakpoint for risk
c. high risk
d. extremely high risk (worst score)

34. Which type of overlay support surface is best for moisture control?

a. rubber
b. plastic
c. gel
d. foam

35. Which of the following characteristics indicates venous insufficiency?

a. pain ranges from intermittent to severe constant
b. pulses are absent or weak
c. brownish discoloration is evident about ankles and anterior tibial area
d. rubor occurs on dependency and pallor on foot elevation

36. Which of the following is a typical example of a peripheral ulcer caused by arterial insufficiency?

a. deep, circular, necrotic ulcer on toe tips
b. irregular ulcer on medial malleolus
c. round ulcer on anterior tibial area
d. irregular ulcer on lateral malleolus

37. When assessing for capillary refill, arterial occlusion is indicated with a refill time of

a. 15 seconds.
b. <2 seconds.
c. >20 seconds.
d. >3 seconds.

38. A pulse graded as 1 on a 0 to 4 scale of intensity could be described as

a. strong and bounding.
b. weak, difficult to palpate.
c. absent.
d. normal, as expected.

39. Which of the following off-loading measures is usually the MOST effective for treatment of neuropathic ulcers?

a. total contact cast
b. removable cast walkers
c. wheelchairs
d. half-shoes

40. Which of the following is characteristic of Charcot arthropathy (Charcot foot)?

a. severe pain and inflammation
b. high arch and hypersensitivity
c. muscle spasms, increased pain, and inflammation
d. weak muscles, reduced sensation, inflammation, and collapsed arch

41. Which of the following is necessary to manage peripheral lymphedema of the legs?

a. daily diuretics
b. static compression bandaging
c. off-loading
d. bed rest

42. Which measurement must be used to evaluate the safety of static compression therapy to manage edema?

a. capillary refill time
b. venous refill time
c. ankle-brachial index
d. blood pressure

43. Which of the following pharmacological measures is used to maximize perfusion with intermittent claudication?

a. antiplatelet agents, such as Plavix®
b. vasodilators, such as cilostazol (Pletal®)
c. thrombolytics
d. anticoagulants, such as warfarin (Coumadin®)

44. Which of the following may be a subtle indication of infection with arterial insufficiency?

a. fever and chills
b. decrease in necrotic area
c. decreased pain or edema
d. fluctuance of periwound tissue

45. A patient with venous insufficiency requires compression therapy and has Unna's boot applied but must be on bed rest for four weeks. Which action is correct?

a. continue Unna's boot therapy during bed rest, but change 2 times weekly
b. continue Unna's boot therapy, but keep leg elevated
c. discontinue Unna's boot therapy during the bed rest period
d. continue Unna's boot therapy, but change only every 2 weeks

46. When doing the nylon monofilament test, how many test sites should be used?

a. 2
b. 4
c. 8
d. 10

47. The *NEXT* step in wound care for a traumatic wound, such as a dog bite, after stabilizing the patient's condition and stopping bleeding is

a. administer antibiotics
b. administer tetanus toxoid/immune globulin as indicated
c. flush wound with copious amounts of normal saline under pressure
d. scrub wound with povidone-iodine

48. A patient with pemphigus vulgaris has generalized lesions with ulcerations and crusting, causing the patient's skin to adhere to the bed sheets. The patient is mobile and otherwise healthy and is seeking recommendations to self-manage this issue. What should the wound care nurse recommend?

a. ensure bed sheets are always clean and dry
b. set an alarm to turn frequently during the night
c. place a piece of soft plastic over the sheets
d. use an alternating pressure mattress

49. What is the most effective treatment for a fungating neoplastic wound of the breast that is oozing blood from eroded vasculature?

a. charcoal dressing
b. hemostatic dressing and cauterization with silver nitrate
c. cleansing with ionic solution
d. surgical debridement

50. One of the primary treatments for contact dermatitis with an itching, blistering rash is

a. nonadherent dressings.
b. topical corticosteroid.
c. antibiotics.
d. cleansing with povidone-iodine.

51. How many grams of protein per kilogram should the average person with a pressure injury receive each day?

a. 1.25-1.5 g/kg
b. 1.5-2.0 g/kg
c. 2.0-2.5 g/kg
d. 2.5-3.0 g/kg

52. If a patient is about to be discharged home from an acute care hospital unit but has poor insurance coverage and is concerned about the costs of dressing supplies, but best referral is likely

a. community agency.
b. social worker.
c. national charity.
d. faith-based organization.

53. If a patient with a chronic leg wound comes to an appointment and the wound has deteriorated because the patient has been changing the dressing one time weekly instead of every 3 days, the MOST appropriate response is,

a. "Let's talk about how I can help you to adhere to the plan of care."
b. "Your wound is deteriorating because you aren't adhering to the plan of care."
c. "Why didn't you change your dressings according to the plan of care?"
d. "If you don't take care of this wound, you might lose your leg."

54. A toe-brachial index should be assessed rather than the ankle-brachial index for patients with

a. pain on walking.
b. history of atherosclerosis.
c. vascular calcification.
d. hypertension.

55. A patient's transcutaneous oxygen pressure measurement ($TCPO_2$) is 18 mmHg, which indicates

a. adequate oxygenation.
b. slight impairment.
c. equivocal finding.
d. marked ischemia.

56. If a patient scheduled for hyperbaric oxygen therapy presents with a severe upper respiratory infection, the treatment should generally be

a. withheld.
b. given for a shorter period of time.
c. given for a longer period of time.
d. given as usual.

57. If using the PQRST method of pain assessment, an appropriate question to begin the assessment with is

a. "Does the pain move or stay in one place?"
b. "When did the pain start?"
c. "What causes the pain?"
d. "What does the pain feel like?"

58. Excessive collagen production at the site of a wound leads to

a. inflammation.
b. abnormal scarring.
c. Dehydration of the wound
d. rapid healing.

59. Hydrocolloid dressings with silver are appropriate for

a. dry infected wounds.
b. dry clean wounds.
c. infected wounds without heavy exudate.
d. non-infected wounds with mild exudate.

60. Which of the following drugs may impede wound healing?

a. NSAIDs
b. levothyroxine
c. insulin
d. ferrous sulfate

61. Which class of therapeutic compression stockings is appropriate for refractory venous ulcers and lymphedema?

a. class 1: 20-30 mmHg.
b. class 2: 30-40 mmHg.
c. class 3: 40-50 mmHg.
d. class 4: 50-60 mmHg.

62. A patient has been prescribed becaplermin gel (Regranex®) according to standard protocol for wound treatment. How many hours out of 24 should the gel be in place on the wound?

a. 6
b. 12
c. 18
d. 24

63. Which comment by the patient suggests that the patient may benefit from a referral to a nutritionist?

a. "I try to eat my three meals within a 14-hour timespan so that I fast for 10 hours."
b. "I've been eating a vegetarian diet for two years."
c. "I limit my meat intake to 4 ounces daily and eat more fruits and vegetables."
d. "I'm substituting honey for sugar in everything, so my carbohydrate intake is lower."

64. If teaching a caregiver to use pillow bridging to prevent pressure injuries for an immobile patient, how many pillows should be employed?

a. 2
b. 4
c. 5
d. 7

65. When assessing a patient with diabetes, it's important to remember that diabetic patients tend to lose protective sensation after

a. 10-15 years.
b. 8-10 years.
c. 5-8 years.
d. 3-5 years.

66. Which of the following steroid dermatologic agents has the highest potency?

a. hydrocortisone acetate
b. desonide
c. triamcinolone
d. betamethasone dipropionate

67. If a patient with a slow-healing coccygeal wound is having negative pressure wound therapy (NPWT) and the nurse is assessing the wound with the DIME acronym, the M refers to

a. mobility.
b. maceration.
c. moisture balance.
d. malodor.

68. If a patient complains of severe pain during dressing changes and has an analgesic order, the analgesic should generally be administered

a. 60-90 minutes before treatment.
b. 30-60 minutes before treatment.
c. 15-30 minutes before treatment.
d. 5-15 minutes before treatment.

69. Which of the following types of debridement is MOST indicated for a wound with large amounts of unviable tissue and increasing cellulitis?

a. sharp debridement
b. enzymatic debridement
c. wet-to-dry debridement
d. autolytic debridement

70. The MOST accurate method of measuring the size and depth of a wound is a

a. ruler.
b. comparison with known object, such as a coin.
c. photograph.
d. stereophotogrammetry.

71. Undermining most often occurs as the result of

a. friction.
b. shear.
c. direct trauma.
d. direct pressure.

72. The odor of a wound should be assessed

a. before the dressing is removed.
b. before cleaning the wound.
c. after cleaning the wound.
d. at all stages of dressing change.

73. If exudate covers less than two-thirds, but more than one-third of a dressing after it is removed, the amount of exudate would be classified as

a. small.
b. moderate.
c. large.
d. excessive.

74. Moisture-associated skin damage (MASD) most often results in

a. maceration of periwound skin.
b. wound infection.
c. eschar development.
d. undermining.

75. Under CMS regulations, how long must a patient have an unsuccessful trial with static compression therapy before switching to intermittent pneumatic compression therapy?

a. 1 month
b. 2 months
c. 4 months
d. 6 months

76. If the edges of a wound are rolled inward, this may indicate any of the following etiologies EXCEPT

a. infection.
b. dehydration.
c. hypoxia.
d. basement membrane formation.

77. When developing the care plan for a patient, the MOST effective method of prioritizing a list of goals is to

a. review the history and physical.
b. ask the physician.
c. ask the patient.
d. refer to a care plan guide.

78. The initial sign of an infection in a chronic wound is often

a. delayed healing.
b. serosanguinous drainage.
c. purulent drainage.
d. pain.

79. When using the STONES mnemonic to help identify a deep infection, the "O" stands for

a. oxygenation.
b. obesity.
c. occlusion.
d. os (bone).

80. When applying a lidocaine 2% soak to a wound, how long should the saturated gauze be left in place prior to debridement of the wound?

a. 30-60 seconds
b. 1-2 minutes
c. 3-5 minutes
d. 6-8 minutes

81. Which of the following support surfaces has low moisture retention?

a. air fluidized
b. static flotation (air, water)
c. alternating air
d. foam

82. When assessing venous flow with duplex ultrasound, retrograde flow is classified as abnormal if it persists for

a. more than 0.5 second.
b. more than 1.0 second.
c. more than 1.5 seconds.
d. more than 2 seconds.

83. Hot tub folliculitis is most often caused by

a. *Staphylococcus aureus.*
b. *Escherichia coli.*
c. *Enterobacter.*
d. *Pseudomonas aeruginosa*

84. The use of topical silver-based creams, such as Silvadene®, should be limited to

a. one week.
b. two weeks.
c. three weeks.
d. four weeks.

85. Which of the following is a contraindication for the use of transparent film dressings?

a. the wound has a small amount of exudate
b. the dressing is applied to protect a pressure spot
c. the wound is covered with dry eschar
d. the wound has a suspected bacterial infection

86. Which of the following are the two primary factors that determine how damaging pressure will be to the tissue?

a. duration and magnitude
b. oxygenation and nutrition
c. duration and oxygenation
d. magnitude and nutrition

87. When evaluating support surfaces, what does *immersion* refer to?

a. the thickness of the support surface
b. the duration that a patient can be left in one position on the support surface
c. the depth the patient's body penetrates the support surface
d. the amount of pressure that the support surface can actually support

88. If a patient's wound has developed epibole and a closed edge, what intervention is needed to increase healing?

a. a moist healing environment
b. debridement of the epibole
c. application of topical antibiotics
d. compression therapy

89. Foam mattresses tend to "bottom out" and should be replaced after about

a. 3 months.
b. 12 months.
c. 2 years.
d. 3 years.

90. Which of the following is a contraindication for use of electrical stimulation to promote healing?

a. pacemaker
b. diabetic neuropathy
c. renal disease
d. edema

91. Which of the following is a recommended position for a patient on a horizontal surface?

a. prone position with rotation of 40 degrees to the right or left
b. supine position with rotation of 40 degrees to the right or left
c. supine position with head of bed elevated ≤30 degrees and knees flexed
d. supine position with head of bed elevated ≤35 degree and feet blocked

92. A patient on a continuous or intermittent lateral rotation support surface is at risk for

a. friction injury.
b. shear injury.
c. pressure injury.
d. moisture injury.

93. Lower extremity girth measurement to assess edema should be done at the metatarsal head, both malleoli, and

a. 2, 8, 14, and 18 cm above the lateral malleolus and lower edge of patella.
b. 2, 4, and 8 cm above the lateral malleolus and lower edge of patella.
c. 8 and 16 cm above the lateral malleolus and lower edge of patella.
d. 3, 12, and 18 cm above the lateral malleolus and lower edge of patella.

94. If a diabetic patient has a stage IV sacral pressure injury with undermining from 4-8 o'clock to 1 cm, a heavy volume of exudate, and a bioburden, which of the following dressings is MOST indicated?

a. packing wound with calcium alginate and covering with bordered foam dressing
b. packing wound with silver alginate and covering with bordered foam dressing
c. packing the wound with normal-saline saturated gauze and covered with absorptive dressing
d. packing wound with a wound filler (starch copolymers) and covering with absorptive dressing

95. If an overweight patient's weight is at the upper limit for a specialty mattress, the correct intervention is to

a. consider the patient's weight distribution.
b. utilize the specialty mattress for the patient's weight.
c. utilize a bariatric mattress.
d. utilize the specialty mattress for the patient's weight with additional support surface.

96. When educating a patient with mild cognitive impairment (MCI) about wound care, one way to deal with the communication barrier is to

a. also instruct a caregiver.
b. write everything down.
c. break instructions into small steps.
d. repeat the instructions numerous times.

97. Biologic therapy with maggots is contraindicated with

a. a wound that has not responded to other treatments.
b. infected wound.
c. painful wound.
d. exposed blood vessels.

98. When carrying out limb volume measurements by the circumferential method, measurements are taken on the hand and arm every

a. 4 cm.
b. 6 cm.
c. 10 cm.
d. 14 cm.

99. The Braden scale for risk of developing pressure injuries assesses 6 different areas: sensory perception, moisture, activity, mobility, usual nutrition pattern, and

a. friction and shear.
b. mental status.
c. pain level.
d. risk of fall.

100. If a patient has a total contact cast applied for offloading for a plantar neuropathic foot ulcer, how frequently should the TCC be changed?

a. every 4-5 days
b. every 1-2 weeks
c. every 2-4 weeks
d. every 4-5 weeks

101. When using Doppler ultrasound to evaluate blood flow, at what angle to the skin should the transducer be held?

a. 20 degrees
b. 45 degrees
c. 75 degrees
d. 90 degrees

102. An essential role of fat in the diet is to

a. provide the most available source of energy.
b. serve as a component of antibodies and the immune system.
c. maintain the normal function of the cell membrane.
d. increase the activation of white blood cells at the wound site.

103. When educating a patient with peripheral arterial disease about self-care, which of the following should the patient be advised poses the greatest risk for decreasing circulation?

a. drinking one glass of wine daily
b. smoking cigarettes
c. using cannabidiol (CBD) cream to reduce pain
d. drinking 2 cups of coffee daily

104. The Braden Q scale was designed specifically for which population?

a. pediatric
b. geriatric
c. obstetric
d. disabled

105. If the nurse is teaching a hearing-impaired patient to do dressing changes, and the patient nods the head and appears to understand, which of the following is the MOST effective method of ensuring the patient understands the information?

a. provide information in writing/visual form as well
b. provide instructions to a family member
c. ask the patient if the instructions are clear
d. ask the patient to do a return demonstration

106. If collagenase is being applied to a wound for debridement, the wound's pH must stay within the range of

a. 2-4.
b. 4-6.
c. 6-8.
d. 8-10.

107. If a patient who is malnourished has the following nursing diagnosis on the plan of care, "Imbalanced nutrition, less than body requirements," which of the following is an appropriate desired outcome?

a. provide supplements if diet remains insufficient
b. patient will improve activity level and show increased energy
c. ensure well-balanced healthy diet
d. patient will maintain adequate nutrition evidenced by weight within normal range

108. Which of the following is a contraindication to surgical/sharp debridement of a wound?

a. diabetic neuropathy
b. ischemic tissue
c. underlying infection
d. deep extensive wound

109. The best method of attaching dressings to vascular leg ulcers is

a. paper tape.
b. ACE bandage.
c. liquid adhesive.
d. tube gauze/netting.

110. If a patient has a diabetic ulcer with minimal to moderate exudate and a small amount of eschar that requires debridement, which of the following dressing choices is MOST appropriate for autolytic debridement?

a. gauze
b. hydrogel
c. alginate
d. hydrocolloid

111. Compression of tissue impairs circulation and can result in ischemia and pressure injury when the skin perfusion pressure falls to below

a. 5-10 mmHg.
b. 10-20 mmHg.
c. 30-40 mmHg.
d. 50-60 mmHg.

112. If a patient score 13 total points in the 5 categories of the Norton Plus Pressure Ulcer Scale and checks positive for diabetes, hypertension, and hemoglobin, what is the patient's risk for pressure injuries?

a. high risk
b. moderate risk
c. low risk
d. no risk

113. The 5 basic elements of a skin assessment include (1) temperature, (2) color, (3) moisture, (4) integrity, and (5)

a. pain.
b. turgor.
c. sensation.
d. edema.

114. If the healthcare provider is using the NERDS mnemonic to identify a superficial infection, the "D" stands for

a. Degeneration.
b. Data.
c. Dusky.
d. Debris.

115. If a wound is characterized by a defective matrix and cell debris that are impairing healing, which of the following is the correct intervention?

a. negative pressure wound therapy
b. moisture-balancing dressings
c. antimicrobials
d. debridement

116. Calluses on the bottom of the foot most often occur because of

a. improperly fitted shoes.
b. shoes that are too soft.
c. dampness, such as from excessive perspiration.
d. going barefoot.

117. With the TIME wound bed preparation approach, the "M" stands for

a. mechanical debridement.
b. measure of wound.
c. moisture balance.
d. maintenance of circulation.

118. In a chronic wound, which phase of wound healing is generally prolonged?

a. hemostasis
b. inflammatory
c. proliferative
d. maturation

119. If an older adult was admitted to the hospital with severe malnutrition and pressure injuries and was started on a high protein diet, which of the following laboratory tests is the BEST measure of short-term change in nutritional status?

a. prealbumin
b. albumin
c. transferrin
d. total protein

120. In a wound, a biofilm may take on the appearance of

a. necrosis.
b. slough.
c. serosanguinous discharge.
d. purulent discharge.

Answer Key and Explanations

1. B: A fistula extends under normal tissue away from the wound and connects two structures, such as the wound and an organ or the wound and the skin. Undermining occurs when damaged tissue lies underneath intact skin about the wound perimeter. Tunneling is damaged tissue extending from the wound under normal tissue but not opening to the skin or other structures. An abscess is a collection of purulent material in a localized area, often occurring with a fistula.

2. D: Abscesses often form in conjunction with fistulae. Typical indications include erythema, pain, and swelling above the localized area of the abscess. If the abscess is deep within the tissue or within an internal organ, however, obvious signs of abscess formation may not be evident, and symptoms may be less specific, including general malaise, abdominal pain, chills, fever, lethargy, diarrhea, and anorexia. Additional symptoms may be specific to the site of the abscess; for example, a perirenal abscess may cause flank pain.

3. C: Prealbumin is most commonly monitored for acute changes in nutritional status because it has a half-life of only 2-3 days. Prealbumin decreases quickly when nutrition is inadequate and rises quickly in response to increased protein intake. Protein intake must be adequate to maintain normal levels of prealbumin.

- Normal value: 16-40 mg/dL
- Mild deficiency: 10-15mg/dL
- Moderate deficiency: 5-9 mg/dL
- Severe deficiency: <5 mg/dL

Total protein levels and transferrin levels may be influenced by many factors, so they are not reliable measures of nutritional status. Albumin has a half-life of 18-20 days, so it is more sensitive to long-term protein deficiencies than to short-term deficiencies.

4. A: Proliferation (days 5-20) is characterized by granulation tissue starting to form at the wound perimeter, contracting the wound, and epithelialization, resulting in scar formation. Hemostasis (within minutes) occurs as platelets seal off the vessels and the clotting mechanism begins. Inflammation (days 1 to days 4-6) is characterized by erythema and edema as phagocytosis removes debris. During maturation or remodeling (days 21 plus), scar tissue continues to form until the scar has about 80% of its original tissue strength and the wound closes; the underlying tissue continues to remodel for up to 18 months.

5. B: Eutectic Mixture of Local Anesthetics (EMLA Cream) is applied thickly (1/4 inch) to both the surface of the wound and surrounding tissue, extending about 1/2 inch past the wound. After application, the wound must be covered with plastic wrap for 20-60 minutes to numb the tissue. EMLA cream is effective for about an hour after the wrapping is removed. EMLA can interact with a number of different medications, such as antiarrhythmics, anticonvulsants, and acetaminophen, so medications should be carefully reviewed prior to administration.

6. D: Normal saline is the most appropriate wound-cleansing solution. Antiseptic solutions should be avoided as they may damage granulation tissue and retard healing because they interfere with fibroblast cells necessary for healing of the wound, cause increased pain, and do not significantly reduce overall bacterial load. In heavily-contaminated or necrotic wounds, topical antiseptic solutions, such as dilute povidone-iodine or hydrogen peroxide, may be used for a short period of time to reduce surface bacteria and foul odor.

7. A: A 35-mL syringe with 19-gauge needle provides irrigation pressure at about 8 psi. A squeeze bottle (250 mL) provides about 4.5 psi, but a bulb syringe usually only provides ≤2 psi. Both syringe/catheter and needle size affect irrigant pressure. Pressures <4 psi do not provide adequate wound cleansing, but pressures >15 psi can result in wound trauma.

- 6 mL/19 gauge = 30 psi
- 12 mL/19 gauge = 20 psi
- 12 mL/22 gauge = 13 psi
- 35 mL/21 gauge = 6 psi
- 35 mL/25 gauge = 4 psi

8. C: Perceptions and expressions of pain vary widely from one individual to another, so the most important criterion for evaluating pain is the patient's own report of pain. Cultural differences have a role in how people express pain, with some cultures typically appearing more stoic than others. Using a 1 to 10 pain scale is an effective tool for people who are cognitively alert. If people are not able to report their pain level, then observation of behavior and facial expressions may give clues to their need for pain medication.

9. A: Hypoalbuminemia is likely to have the most negative effect on wound healing. Hypoalbuminemia is an indication of protein malnutrition (kwashiorkor) and may cause delayed wound healing because of inadequate nutrition. A BMI of 20.2 is within normal range (18.5-24.9) and indicates normal weight. A person with a BMI of 29 is overweight, but not obese. Both being underweight (BMI <18.5) and obese (BMI >30) can interfere with the body's ability to heal. BMI alone is not adequate to assess nutritional status or healing ability, and vegan diets can provide adequate nutrition.

10. A: The most definitive method of obtaining a wound specimen for culture and sensitivities is a tissue biopsy. A needle biopsy can also provide an adequate sample in many cases. Swabbing a wound with a sterile applicator often does not provide an adequate sample, because this method obtains material only from the wound surface, which may include both pathogenic agents from the wound and contamination from skin bacteria. The tissue itself must be cultured, not just the discharge.

11. B: Corticosteroids may impair wound healing by interfering with vascular proliferation and epithelialization. The anti-inflammatory effect may interfere with the inflammatory phase of healing by decreasing migration of macrophages and polymorphonuclear leukocytes to the wound, interfering with angiogenesis, and increasing susceptibility to wound infection. Other drugs that may impair healing include vasoconstrictors, NSAIDs, aspirin, colchicine, immunosuppressant's, DMARDS (anti-rheumatoid-arthritis drugs), and anticoagulants. Some drugs appear to promote wound healing, including phenytoin, prostaglandin, and estrogen.

12. B: A burn extending into the dermis with obvious blistering would be classified as a second-degree burn. A first-degree burn is superficial and involves only the epidermis. First and second-degree burns, like other wounds, may also be classified as partial-thickness injuries, because the vessels and glands necessary for healing remain intact. A third-degree burn, also classified as a full-thickness injury, extends through the dermis and into the underlying subcutaneous tissue and may extend through vessels, nerves, muscle and even to the bone.

13. B: The nicotine in cigarettes is a powerful vasoconstrictor and interferes with oxygen transport. The carbon monoxide from smoking displaces oxygen on hemoglobin, decreasing the level of oxygen in the blood. Vasoconstriction reduces delivery of nutrients needed for healing. Peripheral blood flow can be reduced by 50% for up to 60 minutes after smoking a cigarette, and oxygen tension may be reduced for 120 minutes. Additionally, nicotine increases the heart rate and blood pressure, so the heart requires more oxygen to function adequately while receiving less.

14. D: The ankle-brachial index (ABI) examination evaluates peripheral arterial disease of the lower extremities. The ankle and brachial systolic pressures are obtained, and then the ankle systolic pressure is divided by the brachial systolic pressure to obtain the ABI. If the ankle systolic pressure is 90 and the brachial systolic pressure is 120: 90 divided by 120 = 0.75. Normal ABI values fall within the range of 1.0 to 1.1, with lower values indicating decreasing perfusion. A value of 0.75 indicates severe disease and ischemia.

15. D: Transcutaneous oxygen pressure measurement ($TCPO_2$) is a noninvasive test that measures dermal oxygen to show the effectiveness of oxygen in the skin and tissues. A value of >40 mmHg indicates adequate oxygenation for healing. Values of 20-40 mmHg are equivocal findings, and values < 20 mmHg indicate marked ischemia, affecting healing. Two or three different sites on the lower extremities should be tested to give a more accurate demonstration of oxygenation. $TCPO_2$ is often used to determine if oxygen transport is sufficient for hyperbaric therapy.

16. B: Secondary healing (healing by second intention) involves leaving the wound open and allowing it to close through granulation and epithelialization. Primary healing (healing by first intention) involves surgically closing a wound by suturing, flaps, or split or full-thickness grafts to completely cover the wound. Tertiary healing (healing by third intention) is also sometimes called delayed primary closure because it involves first debriding the wound and allowing it to begin healing while open and then later closing the wound through suturing or grafts. Quaternary prevention includes activities to prevent iatrogenic disorders/effects.

17. C: Increased serum sodium and serum osmolality indicate dehydration. Serum sodium measures the sodium level in the blood.

- Normal values: 135-150 mEq/L
- Dehydration: >150 mEq/L

Serum osmolality measures the concentration of ions, such as sodium, chloride, potassium, glucose, and urea, in the blood. Levels increase with dehydration, which stimulates the antidiuretic hormone, resulting in increased water reabsorption and more concentrated urine in an effort to compensate.

- Normal levels: 285-295 mOsm/kg
- Dehydration: >295 mOsm/kg

18. C: Autolytic debridement is effective for small wounds without infection, but it is slower than other types of debridement. Autolytic debridement requires an occlusive or semi-occlusive dressing to create a warm moist wound environment. Any moisture-retentive dressing, such as hydrocolloids, alginate, and hydrogels, and transparent film, can promote some degree of autolytic debridement, but because of drainage and odor, surrounding tissue must be protected with some type of skin barrier to prevent tissue maceration.

19. A: Enzymatic (chemical) debridement requires application of enzymes 1-2 times daily and is most effective for a wound with necrosis and eschar, which must be crosshatched if it is dry. Enzymes include the following:

- Collagenase, applied 1 time daily. Wound pH must remain at 6-8 or the enzyme deactivates. Deactivated by Burrows solutions, hexachlorophene, and heavy metals.
- Papain/urea combinations, applied 1-2 times daily. Wound pH must remain at 3-12. Deactivated by hydrogen peroxide and heavy metals.

20. C: Pain and bleeding indicate that viable tissue is being debrided, so debridement must be discontinued. Only necrotic tissue/eschar should be removed by sharp debridement, removing small layers at a time to prevent injury to viable tissue. Purulent discharge often occurs with an infected wound. While patient fatigue is a concern, positioning the patient for comfort, explaining the procedure, and reassuring the patient may help the patient tolerate continuing the procedure until the wound is adequately debrided.

21. D: Surgical debridement is most commonly used when very large amounts of tissue must be debrided, such as with extensive burns, or when immediate debridement is needed in order to effectively treat a serious wound infection. General anesthesia allows extensive debridement to be done without the patient suffering associated pain and trauma, although postoperative pain is common. One advantage is that most debridement can be done in one procedure. Lasers may also be used for surgical debridement, with pulsed lasers posing less risk to adjacent tissue than continuous lasers.

22. A: In the past, wet-to-dry gauze dressings were frequently used for wound care; however, wet-to-dry dressings have little use in current wound care unless the wound is very small because the gauze adheres to the wound and can disrupt granulation or epithelization. While a whirlpool bath may effectively cleanse debris from a wound, concerns about cross infection have resulted in less frequent use of the whirlpool. Ultrasound may effectively débride wounds. Irrigating a wound with pressurized solution can be effective if the pressure remains in the optimal range, usually 8-12 psi.

23. C: Mupirocin is effective against Gram-positive organisms, such as *Staphylococcus aureus* and MRSA, and is used for treating nasal colonization to decrease risk of wound infection. Cadexomer iodine is effective against a wide range of bacteria, viruses, and fungi and is placed in the wound where beads of iodine swell in contact with exudate, releasing the iodine into the wound. Metronidazole is effective against bacterial infections, such as MRSA. Silver sulfadiazine is often used to treat burns and is effective against Gram-positive organisms, including *Staph*, MRSA, and Strep.

24. B: Contraindications to negative pressure wound therapy include wound malignancy, untreated osteomyelitis, exposed blood vessels or organs, and nonenteric, unexplored fistulas. Negative pressure therapy uses subatmospheric (negative) pressure with a suction unit and a semi occlusion vapor-permeable dressing. The suction reduces periwound and interstitial edema, decompressing vessels, improving circulation, stimulating production of new cells, increasing the rate of granulation and reepithelialization, and decreasing colonization of bacteria. NPWT is used for a variety of difficult-to-heal wounds, especially those that show less than 30% healing in 4 weeks of postdebridement treatment or those with excessive exudate.

25. A: The primary goal in referring a patient for multidisciplinary consultation is to prevent complications. A multidisciplinary team is composed of experts in a number of different fields, collaborating to address the complex problems associated with wound care and underlying pathology. Instead of the serial approach to problem-solving involved in the traditional model of care, where referrals are made in response to problems that arise with little communication among specialists, the multidisciplinary approach attempts to identify potential problems and institute preventive measures at the onset, with all members communicating and sharing information.

26. D: Becaplermin (Regranex®) gel is indicated for treatment of peripheral diabetic ulcers extending into subcutaneous tissue or deeper with adequate perfusion. Application follows debridement and usually about 3 weeks offloading if healing is not adequate. Becaplermin is a growth factor derived from human platelets. It is not approved for use with pressure injuries and stasis ulcers and should not be used with closed (sutured/stapled) wounds. Becaplermin is associated with increased risk of developing malignancy and increased risk of death from existing malignancy.

27. A: Alginates are effective for infected full-thickness wounds with undermining, tunneling, and large amounts of exudate. They are made from brown seaweed and absorb exudate, forming a hydrophilic gel that conforms to the shape of the wound. Hydrocolloids are effective for clean wounds with granulation and minimal to moderate exudate, but they increase the risk of anaerobic infection and hypergranulation. Hydrogels are effective for partial- or full-thickness wounds that are dry or have a small amount of exudate. Hydrogels can be used with necrotic and infected wounds. Semipermeable film is effective over intravenous sites or dry, shallow, partial-thickness wounds.

28. B: The usual hyperbaric oxygen therapy (HBOT) for chronic wounds and lower extremity diabetic ulcers is compression at 2.0-2.4 ATA for 90 minutes daily, with at least 30 treatments. Oxygen toxicity may occur with treatment over 90 minutes. Hyperbaric oxygen therapy (HBOT) is treatment in a high-pressure chamber while breathing 100% oxygen, which increases available oxygen to tissues by 10-20 times, improving perfusion. HBOT results in:

- Hyperoxygenation of blood and tissue
- Vasoconstriction, reducing capillary leakage
- Angiogenesis, because of increased fibroblasts and collagen
- Increased effectiveness of antibiotics needing active transport across cell walls (fluoroquinolone, amphotericin B, aminoglycosides)

29. C: This is a stage III injury. NPIAP stages include:

- Suspected deep tissue injury: purple/reddish discoloration and boggy, mushy, or firm tissue
- Stage I: skin intact with localized non-blanching reddened area, often over bony prominences
- Stage II: abrasion, blister, or slightly depressed area with red/pink wound bed, partial-thickness skin loss, but no slough
- Stage III: deep, full-thickness ulceration that exposes subcutaneous tissue with possible presence of slough, tunneling and undermining without visibility of underlying muscle, tendon, or bone
- Stage IV: deep, full-thickness ulceration with extensive damage, necrosis of tissue extending to muscle, bone, tendons, or joints
- Unstageable: cannot be staged before debridement because of the extent of slough/eschar

30. B: The most common cause of shear is elevation of the bed >30°. Shear occurs when the skin stays in place and the underlying tissue in the deep fascia over the bony prominences stretches and slides, damaging tissue and vessels, which become thrombosed, often resulting in undermining and deep ulceration. Friction against the sheets holds the skin in place while the body slides down the bed, causing pressure and damage in the sacrococcygeal area. The head of the bed should be maintained <30° except for the brief periods when the patient is lifted with a pull sheet or lifting device and turned, at least every 2 hours.

31. A: Support surface material should provide at least one inch of support under areas to be protected when in use to prevent "bottoming out." (Check by placing a hand palm up under the overlay, below the pressure point.) Static support surfaces are appropriate for patients who can change position without increasing pressure to an existing pressure injury. Those needing assistance to move require dynamic support surfaces. Dynamic support surfaces are also needed when static pressure devices provide less than an inch of support.

32. C: The 30° lateral position is better than the 90° side-lying or supine positions because it prevents pressure over bony prominences. Prone (face down) is not comfortable for most patients and requires careful positioning. Devices such as pillows or foam should be used to correctly position patients so that bony prominences are protected and not in direct contact with each other. Patients should not be positioned on existing pressure injuries. Goals for repositioning and a turning schedule of at least every 2 hours should be established for each individual and documented.

33. C: A Braden score of 12 indicates high risk. The Braden scale rates 5 areas (sensory perception, moisture, activity, mobility, and usual nutrition pattern) with a 1 to 4 scale and one area (friction and shear) with a 1 to 3 scale. Lower scores correlate with increased risk. The scores for all six items are totaled, and a risk is assigned according to the number.

- 23 (best score): excellent prognosis with very minimal risk
- ≤16: breakpoint for risk of pressure injury (will vary somewhat for different populations)
- 12-14: high risk
- 6 (worst score): very poor prognosis with strong likelihood of developing pressure injury

34. D: Foam overlays provide the best moisture control for preventing moisture damage to skin. Some materials, such as rubber, plastic, or gel, may increase perspiration and moisture, while some porous materials, including some types of foam, may reduce perspiration. Foam varies considerably in density and indentation load definition (ILD). ILD is the number of pounds of pressure needed to make an indentation in a 4-inch foam of 25% of its thickness, using an indentation of 50 square inches. Foam can be closed-cell (resistant) or open-cell (viscoelastic). Open-cell foam is temperature-sensitive, helping it to mold to the body as it reaches the patient's body temperature.

35. C: Venous insufficiency is characterized by hemosiderin staining (brownish discoloration) about the ankles and anterior tibial area. Pain is usually aching and cramping, and peripheral pulses are present. Lipodermatosclerosis occurs in the lower leg area as the tissue becomes fibrotic from fibrin and protein (collagen) deposits, causing the skin to feel waxy and the tissue to harden, with narrowing of the tissue around the ankle compared to proximal tissue above. Venous (stasis) dermatitis is inflammation of the epidermis and dermis, resulting in scaly, erythematous, crusty, weepy, itchy skin, usually in the lower leg (ankle and tibia).

36. A: Arterial ulcers are characterized by painful, deep, circular, often necrotic ulcers on toe tips, toe webs, heels or other pressure areas, with little edema of extremity. Because circulation is impaired, peripheral pulses are weak or absent, and skin is pale, shiny, and cool, with loss of hair on toes and feet and little edema. Nails are thick with ridges. Rubor occurs on dependency, and pallor occurs on foot elevation. Venous ulcers, by contrast, are typically superficial, irregular ulcers on the medial or lateral malleolus and sometimes on the anterior tibial area, with varying pain and moderate to severe edema of extremity.

37. D: A capillary refill time of >3 seconds indicates arterial occlusion. To assess capillary refill, grasp the toenail bed between the thumb and index finger and apply pressure for several seconds to cause blanching. Release the nail and count the seconds until the nail regains normal color. Check both feet and more than one nail bed. Assess venous refill time with the patient lying supine for a few moments and then have the patient sit with the feet dependent. Observe the veins on the dorsum of the foot and count the seconds before normal filling. Venous occlusion is indicated with times >20 seconds.

38. B: A pulse graded 1 would be weak and difficult to palpate. Pulses should first be evaluated with the patient in a supine position and then again with the legs dependent, checking bilaterally and proximally to distally to determine if the intensity of pulse decreases distally. Pedal pulses should be examined at both the posterior tibialis and the dorsalis pedis. The pulse should be evaluated for rate, rhythm, and intensity, which is usually graded on a 0–4 scale.

- 0 – pulse absent
- 1 – weak, difficult to palpate
- 2 – normal, as expected
- 3 – full
- 4 – strong and bounding

39. A: Total contact casts (TCCs) encase the lower extremity in a walking cast that equalizes pressure of the plantar surface. The casts may have windows over pressure injuries to allow observation and treatment. TCC is more successful than other off-loading measures, possibly because people restrict activity more. Removable cast walkers allow patients to remove the casts, but studies show that people only use them 28% of the time, decreasing effectiveness. Wheelchairs allow dependency of using a limb but prevents pressure. Half-shoes may have a high walking heel with the front of the foot elevated off of the ground.

40. D: Charcot arthropathy results from neuropathy that weakens the muscles of the foot and reduces sensation. As muscles supporting the bones weaken, the bones become weak and fracture easily. Because of the lack of sensation, the patient may be unaware of the fracture and continue to walk, causing further deformity. It causes inflammation, swelling, and increased temperature in the foot, but usually no pain. In time, the joint dislocation causes the arch to collapse. Treatment includes:

- Compression bandages for 2-3 weeks
- Total contact or non-weight-bearing cast for up to 9 months
- Gradual weight-bearing after skin has resumed its normal temperature

41. B: Lymphedema is managed with static compression bandaging during the day, providing 40-60 mmHg of pressure. Bandaging may be removed at night if the limb is elevated. Dynamic compression may be used, but it can displace fluid or further damage lymphatics if not monitored carefully. Diuretics do not help. Lymphedema is a dysfunction of the lymphatic system, resulting in a debilitating, progressive disease. Proteins, lipids, and fluids accumulate in interstitial spaces, causing pronounced induration, edema, and fibrosis of tissues, resulting in distention and thick fibrotic skin with orange discoloration (peau d'orange). Scaly keratotic debris collects, and the skin develops cracks and leaks of lymphatic fluid.

42. C: Static compression is contraindicated if the ankle brachial index (ABI) is <0.5. Compression therapy serves as a preventive and therapeutic treatment to eliminate edema. It is contraindicated in those with heart failure or peripheral arterial disease, because it may further impair compromised arterial circulation.

- High-level compression provides therapeutic compression at 30-40 mmHg at the ankle. Some may provide pressure at 40-50 mmHg. ABI should be >0.8.
- Low-level compression provides modified pressure up to 23 mmHg at the ankle. ABI must be >0.5 and <0.8. While this level is less than therapeutic, even low levels of pressure may provide some therapeutic benefit.

43. B: While vasodilators may divert blood from ischemic areas, some, such as cilostazol (Pletal®) or pentoxifylline (Trental®), may be indicated. Vasodilators dilate arteries and decrease clotting and are used for control of intermittent claudication. If medications do not relieve symptoms, surgical intervention, such as bypass grafts, angioplasty, and even amputation (if ischemia is irreversible), may be necessary. Surgery is indicated with ABI <0.5 or >0.5 if the patient fails to respond to medication and lifestyle changes or with intolerable, incapacitating pain.

44. D: Subtle indications of infection with arterial insufficiency include fluctuance (soft, wavelike texture) of periwound tissue on palpation, increased pain in the ischemic limb, or ulcer and/or increased edema, increased area of necrosis, and slight erythema about wound perimeter. Because of the lack of circulation, the normal signs of inflammation and infection may not be evident with arterial insufficiency, so observing for subtle signs of infection is critically important. Prompt identification and treatment is necessary to prevent cellulitis and/or osteomyelitis, which might necessitate amputation.

45. C: Unna's boot (ViscoPaste®) is a gauze wrap impregnated with zinc oxide, glycerin, or gelatin to provide a supporting compression "boot" to support the calf muscle pump during ambulation, so it is not suitable for non-ambulatory patients and should be discontinued during the bed rest period. The bandage must be applied carefully, without tension. It may either be left open to dry or covered with an elastic or self-adherent wrap. The dressings are changed according to individual needs, determined by a decrease in edema, the amount of exudate, and hygiene, with dressing changes ranging from twice weekly to once every other week.

46. D: The nylon monofilament test is evaluated according to how many of 10 test sites the patient is able to detect, with <4 indicative of decreased sensation. To test, use this procedure:

- Ask the patient to indicate when the monofilament pressure is felt.
- Grasp a length of #10 monofilament in the instrument provided.
- Touch the monofilament against the bottom of the foot, and then press the monofilament into the foot until the line buckles.

- Test the great, 3rd, and 5th toes.
- Test the left, medial, and right areas of the ball of the foot.
- Test the right and left of the arch.
- Test the middle of the heel.
- Test the dorsal aspect of the foot.

47. C: Traumatic injuries are usually contaminated, and once the patient is stable and the bleeding is controlled, the wound should be flushed with copious amounts of isotonic normal saline under pressure (8-12 psi), usually 100-200 mL of irrigant per inch of wound. Prophylactic antibiotics may be given for 3-7 days for superficial wounds and up to 14 days with evidence of infection. Tetanus toxoid or tetanus immune globulin may be necessary if vaccination is not current. Animal bites may also require rabies postexposure prophylaxis (PEP).

48. A: Pemphigus vulgaris (PV), an autoimmune disorder causing blistering of both the skin and the mucus membranes (presenting symptom in 50 to 70% of patients), creates burn-like wounds, which may heal slowly or not at all, often starting in the mouth and genital areas. Untreated, the disorder can lead to death. Blisters on skin rupture, causing ulcerations, and those in folds may develop hypergranulation and crusting. Treatment includes corticosteroids, immunosuppressive drugs, and plasmapheresis to remove antibodies. Ensuring that bed sheets are always clean and dry will help keep the patient's skin from sticking to them and prevent the introduction of infection.

49. B: The ulcers of fungating neoplastic wounds bleed as the vasculature erodes, so hemostatic dressings (gel foam, alginates) and cauterization with silver nitrate may be necessary. Using nonadherent dressings or long-term dressing reduces trauma. Charcoal dressings control odor, and ionic cleansers or antiseptics may be used to cleanse the wound. A foam, alginate, or hydrofiber dressing or wound pouch is used to manage exudate. Skin sealants, barrier ointments, and hydrocolloid wafers to anchor tape protect periwound tissue.

50. B: With contact dermatitis, topical corticosteroid is used to control inflammation and itching. Skin should be gently cleansed with water or oatmeal bath and left open without dressings. Antibiotics are needed only if a secondary infection occurs. Caladryl® lotion may relieve itching, and antihistamines may reduce allergic response. Contact dermatitis is a localized response to contact with an allergen, resulting in a rash that may blister and itch. Common allergens include poison oak, poison ivy, latex, benzocaine, nickel, and preservatives, but people may react to a wide range of items, preparations, and products.

51. A: The average person with a pressure injury should receive 1.25-1.5 g/kg per day, but the patient's kidney function should be assessed to determine if the person can tolerate high levels of protein. Protein has important roles in healing, increasing synthesis of collagen and proliferation of epidermal cells. Protein also has immune properties, is a component of antibodies, and takes part in chemical reactions throughout the body. Each gram of protein provides 4 kilocalories.

52. B: If a patient is about to be discharged home from an acute care hospital unit but has poor insurance coverage and is concerned about the costs of dressing supplies, the best referral is likely a social worker. A social worker can help the patient find resources, including community resources, and determine if the patient may be eligible for Medicaid or for manufacturer's patient assistance programs and assist the patient with applying for appropriate programs.

53. A: If a patient with a chronic leg wound comes to an appointment and the wound has deteriorated because the patient has been changing the dressing one time weekly instead of every 3 days, the most appropriate response is, "Let's talk about how I can help you to adhere to the plan of care." This is a non-judgmental response that may encourage the patient to share rather than being defensive. There can be many reasons why a patient doesn't adhere to the plan of care, including inability to pay for supplies.

54. C: A toe-brachial index should be assessed rather than the ankle-brachial index for patients with vascular calcification. If vessels are calcified, then correct measurements are impossible because the vessels cannot be compressed. The vessels in the toe are much smaller so the calcification that is present rarely encircles the entire vessel, so the vessel can be compressed for testing. A pressure of at least 50 mmHg is required for healing; 20-30 mmHg indicates vascular compromise, which can impair healing of lesions.

55. D: Marked ischemia. Transcutaneous oxygen pressure measurement ($TCPO_2$) assesses dermal oxygen and is used to determine if oxygenation is sufficient for hyperbaric oxygen treatment, to determine the optimum site for amputation, and to determine the degree of hypoxia in tissues. Contact gel and electrodes are applied to the lower extremities to determine variations in oxygen tension. Test results:

- >40 mmHg adequate oxygenation for healing
- 20-40 mmHg equivocal finding
- <20 mmHg marked ischemia, affecting healing

56. A: If a patient scheduled for hyperbaric oxygen therapy presents with a severe upper respiratory infection, the treatment should generally be withheld because an upper respiratory infection increases the risk of developing barotrauma. URIs are considered a relative contraindication. Other relative contraindications include lung disorders (such as COPD and asthma), high fever, pregnancy, seizure disorders (the threshold for seizures may be lowered), medical devices (may malfunction unless approved for hyperbaric oxygen therapy), abnormalities of the eustachian tube, and claustrophobia.

57. C: "What causes the pain?"

PQRST Method of pain assessment

P	Perception/Provoking factors	What causes the pain? What relieves the pain or makes it worse?
Q	Quality of pain	What does the pain feel like? Would you describe the pain as sharp, dull, stabbing, shock-like, aching, burning?
R	Radiation	Does the pain move or stay in one place?
S	Severity	Can you rank the pain on a scale of 1 to 10?
T	Time (onset and duration)	When did the pain start? How long did it last?

58. B: Excessive collagen production at the site of a wound leads to abnormal scarring. This often results from dehydration of the tissue, which stimulates keratinocytes to produce cytokines. These in turn cause fibroblasts to release collagen. Hydrating agents, such as silicone sheets/gels (dimethicone) should be applied to the scar to maintain hydration and prevent transepidermal water loss (TEWL). TEWL increases when the barrier function of the skin is impaired. TEWL can be affected by both intrinsic factors (inadequate intake of fluids, fever) and environmental factors (temperature, humidity).

59. D: Hydrocolloid dressings with silver are appropriate for non-infected wounds with mild exudate. The silver requires exudate in order to be released, but hydrocolloid dressings are inappropriate with heavy exudate or for infected wounds. The silver has antimicrobial action. The hydrocolloid dressing can be left in place for up to a week before changing the dressing, but this may depend on the amount of exudate. Hydrocolloid dressings with silver deactivate enzymatic agents used for debridement.

60. A: Medications that may impede wound healing include NSAIDs and steroids. Steroids, especially, have a negative effect on healing and may increase the risk of skin breakdown. Patients' medication lists should be reviewed if wound healing is slow. Other drugs that may impede healing include anticoagulants, antibiotics (some classes), anti-angiogenesis agents, methotrexate, colchicine, and vasoconstrictive agents. Some drugs, such as levothyroxine, phenytoin, insulin, estrogen, and ferrous sulfate may improve wound healing.

61. C: Class 3 (40-50 mmHg) therapeutic compression stockings are appropriate for refractory venous ulcers and lymphedema. Compression stockings may be used to prevent ulcers after edema is controlled or with existing ulcers when edema recedes. The stockings come in many sizes and colors and may extend from the foot to the knee or the groin. The stockings must be fitted properly and have the correct level of compression:

- Class I*:* 20-30 mmHg (varicose veins)
- Class 2: 30-40 mmHg (venous ulcers and prevention)
- Class 3: 40-50 mmHg (refractory venous ulcers and lymphedema)
- Class 4: 50-60 mmHg (lymphedema)

62. B: If a patient has been prescribed becaplermin gel (Regranex®), a growth factor derived from platelets, according to standard protocol for wound treatment, the gel should be left in place for 12 out of 24 hours. The wound is cleansed with saline or water, becaplermin gel is applied, and the wound is covered with a saline-moistened gauze dressing. After 12 hours, the dressing and gel is removed, and the wound is covered with saline-moistened gauze only for the remaining 12 hours.

63. D: The comment by the patient that suggests that the patient may benefit from a referral to a nutritionist is, "I'm substituting honey for sugar in everything, so my carbohydrate intake is lower." In fact, a teaspoon of honey has 7 g of carbohydrate compared to about 5 g per teaspoon of sugar. Sugar, honey, and maple syrup all metabolize in a similar manner in the body and should be limited in a healthy diet.

64. C: teaching a caregiver to use pillow bridging to prevent pressure injuries for an immobile patient, five pillows should be employed:

- First under legs to elevate the heels
- Second between the ankles
- Third between the knees
- Fourth behind the back
- Fifth under the head

In some cases, a small pillow may also be placed under the upper arm for comfort when the patient is positioned on the side.

65. A: When assessing a patient with diabetes, it's important to remember that diabetic patients tend to lose protective sensation after 10-15 years; therefore, patients may not feel a lesion and need to be educated about the importance of examining the feet daily, avoiding going barefoot, wearing well-fitting shoes, and seeing a physician if any abnormality is noted. Patients may also begin to develop neuropathic pain or numbness, which can interfere with recognition of skin lesions.

66. D: Betamethasone dipropionate (Diprolene®) has ultra-high potency as a steroid dermatologic agent. Hydrocortisone acetate and Desonide have low potency while triamcinolone has medium potency. Betamethasone, which comes in ointment, cream, and lotion forms, is used for lesions that are non-responsive to lower-level corticosteroids, as well as for lichen planus and insect bites. Betamethasone is typically applied twice daily.

67. C: If a patient with a slow-healing coccygeal wound is having negative pressure wound therapy (NPWT) and the nurse is assessing the wound with the DIME acronym, the D refers to debridement, I to infection/inflammation control, M to moisture balance and E to wound Edge preparation. Eschar must be removed from the wound prior to NPWT, and infection must be cleared. The moisture balance should be evaluated with each dressing change. If too dry, the wound healing will slow and eschar may form, so the negative pressure should be reduced or type of packing changed. If the wound is too moist, maceration may occur, and the pressure may need to be increased.

68. B: If a patient complains of severe pain during dressing changes and has an analgesic order, the analgesic should generally be administered 30-60 minutes before treatment to ensure that the medication has peaked. Soaking a dressing with water or NS may help to loosen it if it is adhering to the wound surface. The nurse should note any signs of infection, which generally increases wound pain, and clean the wound of exudate and any debris to reduce the bioburden.

69. A: The type of debridement most indicated for a wound with large amounts of unviable tissue and increasing cellulitis is sharp debridement because this is the fastest method of converting a necrotic wound to a clean wound and allows for better assessment and treatment of the cellulitis. Sharp debridement may be done as a one-time surgical procedure or as a series of sequential debridements. In some cases, laser debridement (considered a form of surgical debridement) may be done if the patient is not a candidate for operative debridement.

70. D: The most accurate method of measuring the size and depth of a wound is stereophotogrammetry (SPG), which creates images and measurements through the use of a digital camera and computer software. The software calculates the size. If measuring manually, a ruler should be used that measures in mm and cm, and the wound size should not be assessed by comparison with known objects, such as a coin.

71. B: Undermining most often occurs as the result of shear or when the surface opening of the wound is smaller than the damage under the surface. Undermining is often documented according to a clock face, "Undermining from 1-3 o'clock, extending 0.75 cm." A thorough description of the undermining should include how far it extends under the tissue and which areas have the most extensive undermining.

72. C: The odor of a wound should be assessed after the dressing is removed and the wound is cleaned because some wound treatments and dressings develop a malodor that may be mistaken for infection. Some infections have a distinctive odor. *Proteus*, for example, has an ammonia-like smell; *Pseudomonas aeruginosa*, a grape-like or sweet odor; and *Escherichia coli*, a floral odor.

73. B: If exudate covers less than two-thirds of a dressing after it is removed, the amount of exudate would be classified as moderate. If the drainage covers less than a third of the dressing, it is classified as a small amount. A large amount is drainage that covers more than two-thirds of the dressing. The amount of exudate provides important information about the condition of the wound and the patient's general condition.

74. A: Moisture-associated skin damage (MASD) most often results in maceration of periwound skin. MASD usually results from wound changes that cause excessive exudate or inadequate dressings to absorb the amount of exudate. With maceration, the skin becomes soft and irritated and often takes on a white, water-logged appearance. Skin barriers and more absorptive dressings, such as alginates, are indicated to better manage exudate.

75. D: Under CMS regulations, a patient must have an unsuccessful trial with static compression therapy for 6 months before switching to intermittent pneumatic compression (IPC) therapy. IPC may also be used if a patient is immobile. IPC devices are used on the lower leg or plantar area of the foot. IPC devices have a garment and a pneumatic pump that inflates the garment. Intermittent inflations occur segmentally up the leg, increasing venous return.

76. D: If the edges of a wound are rolled inward (also known as epibole), this may be caused by a variety of factors including infection, trauma, extreme dehydration, hypoxia, dysfunction of the wound bed, or insufficient basement membrane formation. In this case, the wound edge must be debrided so that the healing process can start again.

77. C: When developing the care plan for a patient, the most effective method of prioritizing a list of goals is to ask the patient what the patient feels is the most important. This patient-focused approach encourages the patient to take an active role in healthcare decisions and shows respect for the patient's autonomy. If the patient is unable to participate, then a parent or caregiver may provide useful insight into what is most important to the patient.

78. A: The initial sign of an infection in a chronic wound is often delayed healing. Typically, an uninfected healing ulcer should show improvement in 2-4 weeks, so if there is no sign of improvement, a wound culture is indicated. The classic signs of infection—erythema, increased temperature, purulent discharge, and edema—may or may not be present, and it can be difficult to distinguish among a deep infection, contamination, and colonization because the response to infection may be altered.

79. D: When using the STONES mnemonic to help identify a deep infection, the "O" stands for os (bone):

- S: Size is bigger
- T: Temperature has increased
- O: Bone is exposed or prone to exposure
- N: New or satellite areas of tissue breakdown are evident
- E: Exudate, erythema, and or edema are evident
- S: Smell is present

80. C: When applying a lidocaine 2% soak to a wound, the saturated gauze should be left in place prior to debridement of the wound for 3-5 minutes. The wound should be thoroughly cleansed with water, saline, or a wound cleaning solution before the gauze, saturated with 5-10 mL of lidocaine, is applied to cover the wound and periwound tissue. Before beginning debridement, the wound should be checked to ensure that it is thoroughly anesthetized.

81. A: Air fluidized and low air loss support surfaces have low moisture retention. Air-fluidized (high air loss) beds are special bed systems in which silicone beads are contained in a bathtub-like frame. There is a high flow of air through the beads. As the air flows through the beads, it "fluidizes" them so that they move, and provide support and redistribution of pressure in much the way water does. The air-fluidized bed is most commonly used for patients with multiple pressure injuries, making positioning to avoid pressure on these injuries very difficult.

82. A: When assessing venous flow with duplex ultrasound, retrograde flow is classified as abnormal if it persists for more than 0.5 second. Various factors, such as trauma or thrombosis, may result in retrograde flow (reflux), which increases hydrostatic pressure and may cause veins to dilate and capillaries to burst. Retrograde flow occurs when the valves are impaired and the flow of blood is reversed when the patient is sitting or standing. Treatment generally includes the use of compression stockings to increase blood flow.

83. D: Hot tub folliculitis is most often caused by *Pseudomonas aeruginosa*. Pruritic pustular lesions usually occur within 1-4 days of exposure to contaminated water in a hot tub. Some patients may have flu-like symptoms in addition to the rash. Generally, the rash is self-limiting within about a week, but persistent or severe infections may require topical or oral antibiotics (such as ciprofloxacin for 5 days), especially in patients who are neutropenic.

84. B: The use of topical silver-based creams, such as Silvadene® (which contains silver sulfadiazine), should be limited to two weeks. Silver sulfadiazine is used to treat second- and third-degree burns and has been found to be effective in reducing bacterial levels. Use should be of limited duration because extended use may increase the risk of resistant bacteria. Additionally, studies have shown that bacterial levels usually decrease markedly within one week.

85. D: A contraindication to the use of transparent film dressings is when the wound has a suspected bacterial or fungal infection. Transparent film dressings should also be avoided with third-degree burns, moderate to heavy exudate, fragile skin, and skin at risk for periwound maceration. Transparent film can be used when a wound has no or minimal exudate or dry eschar that will be debrided and to help secure other dressings in place over the wound.

86. A: The two primary factors that determine how damaging pressure will be to the tissue are duration (the length of time the pressure occurs) and magnitude (the amount of pressure exerted). As the magnitude increases, the duration must decrease in order to protect the tissue. Pressure points of greatest concern include the sacrum, greater trochanters, ischial tuberosities, heels, and scapula. However, other areas may also be at risk, such as ears, depending on the position of the patient.

87. C: When evaluating support surfaces, *immersion* refers to the depth the patient's body penetrates the support surface and is a factor is the dispersal of pressure. For example, on a hard surface, the pressure is more localized to pressure points, but on a softer surface that allows greater immersion, the pressure is more dispersed. However, immersion is different from compression. If a support surface is too compressed, then the pressure localizes, regardless of the type of support surface.

88. B: If a patient's wound has developed epibole and a closed edge the intervention that is needed to increase healing is debridement of the epibole, which may be done surgically or conservatively, such as with silver nitrate. In some cases, vigorous scrubbing of the epibole with gauze or monofilament fiber dressings may be sufficient to open the tissue. Epibole occurs when upper epidermal cells proliferate over lower epidermal cells rather than across the open wound, causing a rolled edge to occur.

89. D: Foam mattresses tend to "bottom out" and should be replaced after about 3 years of use because foam begins to degrade over time. Two types of foam support surfaces are available: elastic and viscoelastic. Some are permeable (open-cell) to fluid and gas, and others are impermeable (closed cell). Support surfaces are often comprised of layers of different densities of foam and different configurations. Foam seat cushions, for example, may be flat, contoured to fit the shape of the person's buttocks, segmented, or cut out.

90. A: Electrical stimulation should be avoided with electronic implants, such as pacemakers, which may be negatively affected. Electrical stimulation is also contraindicated with malignancy, osteomyelitis, and presence of topical substances containing metal ions. A commonly used device provides high voltage pulsed current (HVPC) with pulse rate of 50-120 pps, peaks of 5-20 microsecond phase duration, voltage between 100 and 500 V, and amplitude between 80 and 200 V for wound healing. Pulse rate varies according to the targeted phase of healing: 30 pps during inflammatory stage and 100-150 pps during other phases. HPVC effectively increases blood flow and reduces edema and bacterial load.

91. C: A recommended position for a patient on a horizontal surface is supine with the head of the bed elevated ≤30 degrees and the knees flexed or the feet blocked. Patients may also be positioned prone or supine with rotation of 40 degrees to the right or left. Regardless of the position, the heels should be supported by pillows to reduce pressure on the heels and pillows may be placed between the knees if rotated to the side.

92. B: A patient on a continuous or intermittent lateral rotation support surface, which moves the patient about a longitudinal axis from side to side, is at risk for shear injuries every time their position is changed. Therefore, the patient must be carefully positioned and supported to prevent the development of pressure injuries or the worsening of existing injuries. Lateral rotation support surfaces are often used for obese patients that are difficult to turn, but the support surfaces typically have a weight capacity, which may vary from 350-1000 pounds.

93. D: Lower extremity girth measurement to assess edema should be done at the metatarsal head, both malleoli, 3, 12, and 18 cm above the lateral malleolus and the lower edge of the patella. Measurement should be done distal to proximal and on both the left and right sides. Lower extremity girth measurement can provide accurate evaluation of changes in edema. The other method of assessment is volumetric measurement, which utilizes a tank and water displacement to determine the amount of edema.

94. B: If a diabetic patient has a large (7 x 3 x 1.5 cm) chronic stage IV sacral pressure injury with undermining from 4-8 o'clock to 1 cm, a heavy volume of exudate, and a bioburden, the dressing that is most indicated is packing the wound with silver alginate and covering with bordered foam dressing. The silver alginate is indicated because of the volume of exudate and the bioburden, as silver has antimicrobial properties. The dressing will need to be changed on a daily basis.

95. A: If an overweight patient's weight is at the upper limit for a specialty mattress, the correct intervention is to consider the patient's weight distribution. If the patient's weight is evenly distributed, then the specialty mattress for the patient's weight is appropriate, but if the distribution is uneven—for example if the patient has very large hips—then a better choice is a bariatric mattress because the patient may bottom out on the weight-appropriate mattress.

96. C: When educating a patient with mild cognitive impairment (MCI) about wound care, one way to deal with the communication barrier is to break instructions into small steps because carrying out actions that require a number of sequential steps can be very confusing to patients with MCI. The healthcare provider should ask the patient what helps them to learn. Some patients may want to take notes while others may need illustrations or written guides.

97. D: Biologic therapy with maggots is contraindicated with exposed blood vessels because the maggots may cause the vessels to bleed. Maggots debride the wound because they secrete proteolytic enzymes as well as cytokines and growth factors. Maggot therapy is typically reserved for wounds that have not responded well to other therapies because patients often object to the use of maggots, which are usually left in the wound for about 48 hours. The maggots must be secured to the wound with a special "maggot cage" and gauze that allows air to circulate because lack of air will kill the maggots.

98. A: When carrying out limb volume measurements by the circumferential method, measurements are taken on the foot and leg every 10 cm with the foot in dorsiflexion position and on the hand and arm every 4 cm with the hand flat. The two other methods of limb volume measurements include water displacement (inserting a limb into a container with a measured volume of water and then measuring the overflow) and Perometer® (using an infrared laser system and software to calculate limb volume).

99. A: Friction and shear. Braden scale:

Sensory perception	(1) Completely limited, (2) very limited, (3) slightly limited, (4) no impairment
Moisture	(1) Constantly moist, (2) very moist, (3) occasionally moist, (4) rarely moist
Activity	(1) Bed, (2) chair, (3) occasional walk, (4) frequent walk
Mobility	(1) Immobile, (2) limited, (3) slightly limited, (4) no limitations
Usual nutrition pattern	(1) Very poor, (2) inadequate, (3) adequate, (4) excellent
Friction and shear	(1) Problem (skin frequently slides down sheets and needs help to move), (2) potential problem (skin slides somewhat during moves, needs assistance, (3) no apparent problem

100. B: If a patient has a total contact cast (TCC) applied for offloading for a plantar neuropathic foot ulcer, the TCC should be changed every 1-2 weeks. With the TCC, healing usually occurs within 6-8 weeks, primarily because it forces the patient to carry out offloading since it rests and immobilizes the area of the lesion. However, the cast may be uncomfortable and makes bathing difficult, so removable cast walkers are often utilized instead.

101. B: When using Doppler ultrasound to evaluate blood flow, conductive gel is placed on the end of the transducer or on the skin and the transducer is then held at approximately a 45-degree angle to the skin (pointing towards the patient's head, which can be anywhere from 30 to 60 degrees). The pulse is counted, noting the intensity, and a marking pen is used to mark the site where the pulse is heard. The echo is at a higher frequency when blood flow is in the direction of the transducer and lower frequency when it is in the opposite direction (representing the Doppler effect/frequency shift).

102. C: An essential role of fat in the diet is to maintain the normal function of the cell membrane, permitting fat-soluble substances (such as vitamins A, D, E, and K) to move in and out of the cell. Fats can also serve as a source of energy when carbohydrates are deficient. Stored fat in the tissues provides insulation and protection against heat and cold. Fat provides 9 kcal/g compared to 4 kcal/g for proteins and carbohydrates.

103. B: When educating a patient with peripheral arterial disease about self-care, the patient should be advised that smoking cigarettes poses the greatest risk for decreasing circulation because the nicotine serves as a vasoconstrictor. With each cigarette, the smoker absorbs about 1 mg of nicotine, although this can vary among patients because of genetic differences and racial differences. Vaping and other smokeless tobacco products (such as chewing tobacco) also pose a risk to patients.

104. A: The Braden Q scale was designed specifically for the pediatric population. The scale is similar to the Braden scale although every category is scored from 1 (worst) to 4 (normal) and the descriptions are age appropriate. The categories include mobility, activity, sensory perception, moisture, friction/shear, and nutrition. The last category does not appear in the adult Braden scale and is tissue perfusion and oxygenation. This category is scored based on MAP, hemoglobin, and oxygen saturation.

105. D: If the nurse is teaching a hearing-impaired patient to do dressing changes, and the patient nods the head and appears to understand, the most effective method of ensuring the patient understands the information is to ask the patient to do a return demonstration. While presenting the information in more than one form (spoken and visual) is also helpful, some patients are unable to read or to follow written directions well, and patients may state that they understand even when they do not.

106. C: If collagenase is being applied to a wound for debridement, the wound's pH must stay within the range of 6-8 because otherwise inactivation will occur. Other substances that may inactivate the enzyme include Burrows solution, heavy metal ions, and hexachlorophene. If papain/urea compounds are utilized for enzymatic debridement, the pH must remain between 3 and 12, and heavy metal salts and hydrogen peroxide may inactivate the enzymes.

107. D: A desired outcome for a patient should clearly reflect the nursing diagnosis. Therefore, if the nursing diagnosis is, "imbalanced nutrition—less than body requirements," the appropriate desired outcome is "Patient will maintain adequate nutrition evidenced by weight within normal range." A number of different outcomes may be listed under "evidenced by." Nursing interventions, such as "provide supplements..." are part of the plan of care and distinct from desired outcomes.

108. B: Ischemic tissue is a contraindication to surgical/sharp debridement because this indicates that the blood supply is inadequate for healing. Other contraindications include malignant lesions (because debridement may spread cancer cells), clotting disorders (anticoagulation is a relative contraindication), immunocompromise, and unstable medical condition. Surgical debridement is primarily used for wounds with an underlying infection, such as cellulitis or sepsis, when the need for debridement is urgent.

109. D: The best method of attaching dressings to vascular leg ulcers is tube gauze/netting, which holds the dressings in place but does not apply excessive pressure on the wound, because it's important to avoid any type of adhesive since the skin is likely to be friable. Adhesives may cause stripping of the skin and further ulceration. If adhesives must be used, silicone adhesives are likely to cause the least skin irritation.

110. D: If a client has a diabetic ulcer with minimal to moderate exudate and a small amount of eschar that requires debridement, the most appropriate dressing choice is a hydrocolloid (such as DuoDERM®, Exuderm®, and Replicare®). Hydrocolloids form a gelatinous mass that keeps the wound hydrated and provides an environment in which autolytic debridement can occur. Hydrocolloids can be used with wounds that have minimal to moderate exudate.

111. C: Compression of tissue impairs circulation and can result in ischemia and pressure injury when the skin perfusion pressure falls to below 30-40 mmHg. Normal skin perfusion pressure may range from 50-100 mmHg. Skin perfusion pressure, which measures blood flow to a wound, may be assessed by applying sensors that detect oxygen about the wound in a normal room environment. The test may also be conducted in a hyperbaric chamber with the patient breathing 100% oxygen to determine if the oxygen content increases with hyperbaric oxygen treatment.

112. A: Score of ≤10 is high risk and 11-15 moderate risk on the Norton Plus Pressure Ulcer scale. Each category (physical condition, mental state, activity, mobility, and incontinence) is score from 1 (worst) to 4 (normal). A one-point deduction is made for each of the following categories for which the patient is positive: diabetes, hypertension, hematocrit (<41% for males and <36% for females), hemoglobin (<4 g/dL for males and <12 g/dL for females), albumin level (<3.3 g/dL, fever (>99.6 °F/37.6 °C), polypharmacy (5 or more), and change in mental status to confused/lethargic within 24 hours. Thus, the patient's initial score was 13, minus 3 points for positive findings of diabetes, hypertension, and hemoglobin for a total score of 10.

113. B: The 5 basic elements of a skin assessment include:

1. Temperature: Normally warm to the touch. Cool may indicate impaired circulation, and hot may indicate inflammation or infection.
2. Color: Varies according to ethnicity, but pallor may indicate impaired circulation, while hyperpigmentation/hypopigmentation may indicate impaired circulation, disease or skin condition (altered melanin deposition).
3. Moisture: May vary from dry to moist, depending on general condition and skin disorders.
4. Integrity: Should be intact and free from open areas.
5. Turgor: Pinched skin should return to normal shape rapidly. Turgor may slow with dehydration and aging skin.

114. D: Debris. NERDS mnemonic to identify a superficial infection:

- N: Non-healing wound is present.
- E: Exudate is present from the wound.
- R: Red and bleeding surface granulation tissue is evident.
- D: Debris includes yellow or black necrotic tissue on the surface of the wound.
- S: Smell or malodor is present from the wound.

115. D: If a wound is characterized by a defective matrix and cell debris that are impairing healing, the correct intervention is debridement, which may be carried out episodically or continually, depending on the condition of the wound. Various methods of debridement may be utilized: autolytic, biological, sharp, mechanical, or surgical. The goal is to restore the wound base so that there is viable tissue that can begin the healing process.

116. A: Calluses on the bottom of the foot most often occur because of improperly fitted shoes, which cause the patient's weight to be unevenly distributed. As calluses thicken, they may begin to crack and fissure, causing pain and discomfort. Treatment includes soaking, filing or with pumice stone, and applying moisturizer. In some cases, inserts may be necessary to better distribute weight.

117. C: TIME wound bed preparation approach:

- **T:** Tissue nonviable or deficient: Carry out debridement.
- **I:** Infection/Inflammation: Administer topical/systemic antimicrobials, anti-inflammatories, and/or protease inhibitors.
- **M:** Moisture balance: Apply moisture-balancing dressings/therapy.
- **E.** Edge margin non-advancing or undermined: Utilize adjunctive therapies, bioengineered skin, debridement, and/or skin grafts.

118. B: In a chronic wound, the inflammatory phase is generally prolonged because of the presence in the wound of neutrophils, which produce proinflammatory cytokines. As new tissue forms, it tends to become degraded through the action of proteinases. Most chronic wounds have full-thickness loss of tissue, resulting in the absence of the basement membrane to which epithelial cells generally attach, making epithelialization a more complex and lengthy process. Chronic wounds are also susceptible to the growth of biofilms, which retard healing.

119. A: Prealbumin is the laboratory test that is the best measure of short-term change in nutritional status because it has a half-life of just 2-3 days. Prealbumin is a good measurement because it quickly decreases when nutrition is inadequate and rises quickly in response to increased protein intake. Protein intake must be adequate to maintain levels of prealbumin. Prealbumin is necessary for transportation of both thyroxine and vitamin A throughout the body.

- Normal value: 16-40 mg/dL
- Mild deficiency: 10-15mg/dL
- Moderate deficiency: 5-9 mg/dL
- Severe deficiency: <5 mg/dL

120. B: In a wound, a biofilm may take on the appearance of slough, so it may be a challenge to differentiate the two, although a biofilm tends to have a shinier and more gel-like appearance from the extracellular polymeric matrix that encloses the biofilm. In fact, the biofilm causes a chronic inflammation that results in increased permeability of vessels and increased exudate, leading to the production of slough, so the presence of slough may be an indication that a biofilm is present. Treatment includes debridement and dressings and topical antibiotics to prevent reformation of the biofilm.